RAISING LEADERS

*An Actionable Guide to Nurture Confidence, Resilience,
and Leadership in Your Teen Through Effective
Communication, Empathy, and Faith Based Parenting*

Joshua Nussbaum

Dedication

To Noah Foster Nussbaum,

You are not just the impetus for and focal point of this book, you are my inspiration. You are the reason I am the man I am today. You are the greatest source of pride (and comedy) in my universe. My best student and most profound teacher. My best friend and my son. I love you with all my heart and soul.

To Heidi,

For giving me the greatest gift, I could never have known to ask for; our son.

Rest In Peace.

To Parents,

May you:

HOLD, but don't baby,

ADMIRE, but don't embarrass,

GUIDE, but don't control,

RELEASE, but don't abandon.

Foreword

As parents, educators, or mentors, we have been entrusted with a unique privilege and responsibility—the task of shaping the next generation of leaders. Our role extends far beyond imparting knowledge and skills; it involves guiding teenagers on a transformative journey that empowers them to positively impact the world. This book is a compass for all those who embrace this noble mission and seek to inspire and nurture the potential within young minds.

Contents

Introduction

In the beginning, God made teenagers, and lo, parents did despair:

Welcome to "Raising Leaders: An Actionable Guide to Nurture Confidence, Resilience and Leadership in Your Teen Through Effective Communication, Empathy and Faith Based Parenting" the book that promises to turn your kid into the next Elon Musk... or at least get them to stop rolling their eyes at you.

We want our kids to be successful, happy, and fulfilled. Still, we often forget that leadership skills are essential to achieving those goals. We focus so much on getting them good grades and ensuring they eat their veggies (or, in our house, their protein) that we forget to teach them how to make tough decisions, communicate effectively, and work well with others. That's where this book comes in.

I'm your host, Joshua Nussbaum, and I'm here to guide you through 15 effective strategies that will help you raise a confident, independent, and empathetic young adult.

But don't worry, this isn't going to be some boring lecture about leadership theory. I assure you. We'll be taking a practical approach to raising leaders, with plenty of funny anecdotes and real-life examples to keep things interesting. But listen, I'm not claiming to be an expert of any kind... I'm not a psychotherapist, and I don't have a degree in behavioral sciences. I've never been the host of MTV's "scared straight," where I take troubled youths and scare the shit out of them by taking them to jails in a dramatic attempt to radically scare them into behavioral reformation (or at least not that I can remember).

Hell, I'm not even a parent! OK...Completely kidding on that last one, but how weird would it be if I were actually writing this book with zero personal experience in the field?

I actually AM a parent and a damn dedicated one. I HAVE been through the myriad of the trials and tribulations that come with raising a teenager. I've had the pleasure of dealing with everything from mood swings to fist swings. Messy bedrooms to rebellious streaks. Principle visits and ideological, moral dilemmas. Many of which were my own.

As his father, coach, and confidant, I've also had the joy of watching my son Noah grow into a Brazilian Jiu Jitsu World Champion, and on top of that, a strong, compassionate, funny, communicative, and highly confident young adult with some pretty badass skill sets to boot. This, along with the fact that parenthood has been the single most frustrating, rewarding, challenging, joyful, confusing, and enlightening adventure of my life, are my reasons for writing this book.

I have been miraculously gifted the task of simultaneously sculpting the personality of my best friend while juggling the paradox of supporting his innate strengths and sanding down his pointier edges.

It's a beautiful burden of love from which I derive an unrivaled, unequivocally incomparable amount of pride. For those of you with a more straightforward vocabulary, that was a highly redundant proclamation of my enormous pride in my son. And saying my son is my greatest source of pride is saying a lot because I've lived a pretty damn eventful life with, in my not-so-humble opinion, a shit ton to be proud of.

Which reminds me of the second reason you should listen to me… I AM a leader.

Note: This is where I am supposed to insert that cliche "About the author" blurb. You know, a resume of awe-inspiring accomplishments to gain credibility while doing my best to sound unpretentious so as to not lose the vast quantity of rapport we have built over our extensive time spent together (aka the time it has taken you to read the past 12 paragraphs!). Hey, in TikTok time, that's like a month.

Well, here goes: BLAH BLAH BLAH, Jr Olympics, BLAH BLAH, millionaire by 25…. rabble rabble, hundreds of employees, top 10 podcast, soon to be a bestselling author if you get off your ass and write me a glowing review. Did I mention I'm ravishingly good looking, too? #micdrop.

Of course, I didn't do it alone. I had help from a wealth of experts who came before me and have dedicated their careers to studying leadership and personal development. I suppose, in the words of Mark Twain, I am standing on the shoulders of giants in that sense. (If I'm being perfectly honest, as any great leader should be, I'm not even entirely sure it was Mark Twain that said that. However, I am in a creative flow and can't be bothered to interrupt the proverbial muse to go fact-check a trivial detail that holds no real bearing on the impact of this book or even the point I was making. You have Google, get off my ass.)

Where.were.we? Ah yes, I've had the support of badass family members, and as I write this, a whole load of (shameless plug) RevLabs Pre-Workout. A lot of Pre-Workout.

But enough about me. Let's talk about you. You're here because you want to help your teenager become a leader, and that's an admirable goal. After all, the world needs more leaders, especially now. But how do you do it? How do you raise a kid that doesn't just get pushed around by the world? A person that doesn't get lost in the shuffle of life? How do you raise a teenager that has what it takes to lead? Well, the good news is that it's not rocket science. In fact, some might say it's harder than rocket science. But don't worry, we'll break it down into 15 manageable steps that you can start implementing today.

Let's begin!

Part 1 – Inside Out Leadership (internal growth)

Chapter 1: Don't Screw Up Your Offspring with Your Own Screw-Ups

(aka Setting a Good Example)

"Setting an example is not the main means of influencing others, it is the only means."

- Albert Einstein

I once heard somewhere that Albert Einstein is miscredited with the greatest number of inaccurate quotes he never actually stated. Honestly, it makes me wonder how that guy, we'll call him Shithead Steve, knew that, or if it is even discernably possible to count every historical figure of all time, let alone how many times anybody anywhere misquoted them in any conversation. Seems implausible. In modeling Einstein myself, I conducted an extensive thought experiment on the matter while sitting here. I determined that Shithead Steve was a quack, probably trying to discredit one of the greatest minds of all time out of jealousy and, as the case may be, inadvertently undermining the writing of THE MOST IMPORTANT PRINCIPLE in this leadership book. Well, too bad, Shithead Steve, you've earned your name, Einstein was a badass, and his quote stays.

Over the years raising my son, I have learned a lot about the importance of setting a good example for my kid. Obviously, it's hard, but I believe it's one of the most important things we can do as parents, especially to develop leadership qualities in our children. So, let's dive in and explore the world of setting a good example.

From the moment our children are born, they watch and learn from us. They observe how we interact with the world around us, deal with difficult situations, and treat others. It's our responsibility to model the behavior we want our children to emulate. By setting a good example, we can instill important values and character traits that will help our children automatically become the best version of themselves.

That would mean rule #1, if this book had "Rules", which it doesn't, would be: "If you want your kid to be a leader... you need to be a leader!" Not exactly sure how to make that happen? Fortunately, by reading this book, you're in for a double benefit. While every exercise, strategy, and tip outlined within these pages aims to teach your kids how to develop essential leadership characteristics, they also hold a hidden agenda: they are designed to teach you, the parents.

Read the following pages with the meta frame or subtext of "IF IT IS TO BE, IT'S UP TO ME! And therefore, I will practice what I intend on preaching... leadership included".

One of my favorite stories about setting a good example (or the lack thereof) is when my son caught me sneaking a cookie before dinner. I think he was six. He looked up at me with those big, innocent eyes that he was exuding purposefully to exacerbate the level of guilt he intended to inflict and said, "But Dad, you always tell us not to spoil our appetites." And I thought to myself, "God, my kids a dick…" followed shortly by, "But, well played, child. Well played."

In all seriousness, this moment reminded me that our kids are ALWAYS WATCHING us, and not just when we are intentionally trying to teach them something, and we need to be mindful of the example we set for them.

Why Is Setting A Good Example Important In Leadership?

Let's talk about why setting a good example is so valuable in leadership and how it applies to raising teenagers. As a leader, whether in the boardroom, in your community, or at home, you're setting the tone for how others should behave. Suppose you want your team or your teenager to act with integrity, accountability, and respect, well in that case, you need to walk the walk and talk the talk and exude those values in your own life. Because when you lead by example, you're not just telling people what to do, you're showing them how it's done.

When it comes to raising teenagers, setting a good example is especially important because they're at that weird stage of life where they're trying to figure out who they are, how they should act in the world, and how to adult. And if you want your teenager to grow up to be a responsible and respectful adult, you can't just give them a lecture and hope for the best.

Think about it. When your teenager sees you living your life with purpose and integrity, they're gonna be like, "Wow, my parents are actually pretty cool. Maybe I should listen to them once in a while." It's like being the superhero parent they always wanted, without the spandex and cape (unless you're into that, no judgment).

If you want your teenager to be responsible, show them what responsibility looks like; Show up when and where you say you will, pay your bills on time, take care of your responsibilities, and also show them that adulting doesn't have to be a boring snooze fest by adding a touch of humor. To show them how to be respectful, well, treat others with kindness and respect, and they'll pick up on that vibe like a catchy Instagram tune.

Teenagers are like sponges. They soak up everything around them, whether it's good or bad, be the kind of role model you want them to emulate. Show them that life is an adventure and that they can be the hero of their own story.

And hey, I get it. Parenting is hard, and nobody's perfect. We all have our moments of slipping up or acting like goofballs. But that's okay. It's not about being flawless; it's about being authentic. Apologize when you mess up, laugh at yourself, and keep moving forward.

Whether you're a leader in the workplace or a parent at home, setting a good example is one of your most powerful tools. It's a ripple effect - when you lead with authenticity and purpose, you inspire others to do the same.

Here are some quick-shot ways to set a good example:

- **Be consistent, and stay steady like a reliable clock:** If you want your teenager to be a stand-up citizen, model the behavior you want them to adopt consistently rather than just occasionally. And if you want your teenager to be honest with you, ensure you're honest with them too.

- **Show some respect, like you're treating royalty:** Remember, respect is a two-way street, and by valuing and acknowledging your teenager's perspectives, you foster an environment of open communication and mutual understanding that empowers them to thrive as impactful leaders. So, embrace their passions, and listen to your teenager's opinions and ideas, even if they're talking about TikTok dances, or any other interest, and let their voices be heard in the journey of discovery and growth.

- **Communicate like a pro:** Mastering the art of effective communication is essential in guiding teenagers toward becoming impactful leaders. Employing "I" statements and honing active listening skills with dedication and finesse will create a platform for authentic and meaningful dialogues, allowing you to connect with your teenager on a profound level and foster an environment where their ideas and aspirations can flourish.

- **Take responsibility like a captain:** Admit when you're wrong and own up to your mistakes. It's okay to make mistakes, folks! By acknowledging and admitting when we are wrong, and taking ownership of our mistakes, we demonstrate integrity and model the courage needed to learn and grow.

- **Practice self-care:** Like you're a precious avocado that needs protection. Exercise, eat healthy, get some sleep, and practice stress-reduction techniques like meditation or mindfulness. Because parenting can be stressful AF.

- **Remember:** Setting a good example for your teenager is like planting a garden. It takes time, effort, and a whole lot of commitment. But if you consistently model positive behaviors, you can help your teenager bloom into a successful, well-adjusted adult.

We all want our children to grow up to be honest, hardworking, and responsible individuals. The best way to teach them these values, and the values in every chapter of this book for that matter, is by modeling them ourselves. If we want our children to be honest, we need to be truthful in our words and actions. We need to work hard ourselves if we want our children to be hardworking. And if we want our children to be responsible, we must be accountable for our actions.

One of the most important ways I model good behavior for my son is by keeping my word. If I tell my son that we will spend the day at the beach, I make sure we spend the day at the beach. It's important to show our children that we value our commitments and take them seriously. This also teaches our children the importance of keeping their own promises.

We're all superheroes who put our kids first. But here's the thing, if you constantly put yourself down or neglect your own health and well-being, your kids are gonna pick up on that faster than a dog sniffs out a bone. Show your kids that you value yourself and your well-being and be the king or queen of self-love occasionally. Because if you do, you're teaching your teenager to do the same, and showing them the path to be happy, healthy, and prosperous.

Leading By Example: Illuminating The Path To Extraordinary Leadership

Leading by example is a powerful way to build trust and loyalty. When leaders consistently demonstrate integrity, respect, and honesty, people know they can rely on them. They see that they practice what they preach, and that authenticity resonates deeply. Their actions become a source of inspiration and motivation for others to step up and follow suit.

Leadership is about actions, not just words, show others what it means to walk the talk in such a manner that your behavior becomes the guiding light for those around you. It's not about claiming authority or achieving personal goals; it's about inspiring others to be their best selves and creating a positive impact.

Leaders who set a positive example create a culture of excellence and accountability. Their behavior influences the attitudes and work ethic of those they lead. When they embody qualities like dedication, humility, and resilience, others are encouraged to go the extra mile and strive for greatness, spreading positive change throughout an organization, community, or even society as a whole.

When you lead by example, you become a catalyst for transformation and create a better future for everyone involved. Be the person you want others to become.

Ways To Set A Good Example

I'm going to touch on some quick brush leadership qualities to model as "good behavior", it can just as easily be stated as "leadership behavior", all of which will be expounded upon in the coming chapters.

It's essential to communicate with our children. Communication is a vital leadership skill that our children will need as they grow, build relationships, manage emotions and situations, and enter the adult world. By encouraging open and honest communication with our children, we are teaching them to express themselves and communicate effectively with others.

But let's be real for a moment, communication with teenagers can be challenging. They have a knack for tuning us out or responding with one-word answers. That's why finding ways to make communication fun and engaging is a good way to go. For example, I am awesome. While that is unrelated to my previous or forthcoming statements, here is a relevant example of making communication fun and engaging.

My Son and I have a multitude of inside jokes, including me purposefully using modern lingo and deliberately making it sound wrong, "hella cringe while dabbing my way to quoting dank memes that are secretly pretty mid." If you don't know what that means, don't worry. Allow it to remain an unsolved mystery of the ages, or (teen)ages, and make up some traditions of your own, like coming up with a "dad joke of the day" or making gratitude lists if you're not funny enough for the first two suggestions.

We take turns sharing our favorite corny jokes and puns, new hip hop releases, or listening to him break down for me, which rolls went well in Jiu Jitsu class, and where he got his ass kicked. It may seem silly, but it's fun to break the ice and spark conversation. We'll elaborate on this more in the upcoming chapter.

Life, as they say, is like a rollercoaster, full of ups and downs, twists and turns, and a lot of screaming! It's our job to show our children how to handle those twists and turns, those tough times that leave us feeling like we're about to lose our lunch. By teaching our kids how to be resilient and bounce

15

back when life throws a curveball, we give them the tools they need to succeed. Because life can be tough, but so are our kids - they just need a little guidance to help steer them through those rough patches.

I came home one day and found Noah in the kitchen grappling with a complex math problem. It was one of those Isosceles triangle conundrums that you may remember from school - or not, if you're like me and haven't used them since you were at school. Noah was ready to throw in the towel and give up. But instead of handing him the solution on a silver platter (mostly because I didn't have the answer or a silver platter), I sat down beside him, and we tackled that little SOB of a triangle together. We talked about the importance of perseverance when faced with a problem and trying different approaches until we find a solution. It was a valuable lesson for both of us. And it showed my son that it's okay to ask for help and to keep pushing forward, even when things get downright tricky.

As parents, and people, it's wise to acknowledge and learn from our mistakes. None of us are perfect, and we all probably make all kinds of mistakes on at least a semi-regular basis, if not on the daily. But here's the thing, by admitting your mistakes and taking responsibility for them, you're teaching your kids the important life lesson of accountability and integrity. It's like you're giving them a VIP backstage pass to the reality show of life (instead of attempting to exude a perfect exterior). So, next time you mess up (which, let's be honest, will probably be in the next handful of minutes), own up to it like a boss! Because nobody likes a parent who can't admit when they're wrong. Did I say parent? I meant person.

I remember a time when I lost my temper with my son and said something I regretted, in a tone I regretted, using proximity to him (we were nose to nose) that I also regretted. Instead of making excuses or denying my mistake, I sat down with him and apologized. We talked about how taking responsibility for our actions is important, even when it's hard. This was a valuable lesson for both of us, strengthening our relationship. Especially after I had him write me a mandatory 1,000-word thank you letter for apologizing to him. Just kidding, but if you didn't catch that was a joke prior to me telling you so, maybe it's time to look around and shake your body out so your retention percentage increases... seriously, this is important shit here.

Setting a good example for our children is essential. How do we do this? By modeling good behavior, communicating effectively, and teaching valuable life lessons through our actions. And lucky for you, all of this is covered in the chapters and principles of this book, which cleverly disguises itself as a guide to developing leadership skills in your teenager while also helping you improve as a human being and parent (you're welcome). By taking on the challenge of guiding our teens with vigor, sincerity, and humor (very much the same way I am approaching the writing of this book), we can help them become the best version of themselves. This doesn't mean they have to be a millionaire CEO. It means they can lead their lives and lead others in the ways that present themselves, and in the opportunities they seek out as their life journeys unfold.

I once saw a meme that depicted leadership beautifully with two pictures. Picture one had a circle around it with a line through it demonstrating what leadership was NOT. It showed leadership as a guy sitting on a thrown being pulled by a sea of underlings over which he had to constantly crack the whip he was holding.

Picture two was the same sea of people pulling the same sled, but instead of a thrown with a king, they were pulling a pile of presents that said things like "Mutual Success, Making an impact, etc.". Instead of sitting in a thrown, the king or leader was out in front of the sea of people pulling with them.

What this simple, yet metaphorically powerful meme means, is that you are in the trenches (or know what it feels like to be there), pulling or pushing where necessary to accomplish something you, as a team, have set out to accomplish.

Noah knows in his heart of hearts at least the following two facts:

1. He and I are on a team together, NO MATTER WHAT, for as long as we are both here.
2. I will not ask anything of him that I haven't done or am not presently doing myself to advance the team.

These are significant facts for him to have not just heard before, but to have internalized deeply because it massively increases the respect level and willingness our followers (in this case, our kids) will have for us, and whatever guidance we attempt to impart.

Take inventory. Do your kids know and understand what you have gone through physically, emotionally, logistically, and financially to be where you are today? If not, maybe remind them...

Do they know you are on the same team forever and ever and ever, no matter what? If NOT, teach them. If so, great! Find a way to continuously reinforce it.

When Noah was born, I was a scared, clueless, broke Junior at San Diego State University. Feeling unable to express myself adequately to anybody face to face, I wrote him a letter, which I decided to give him on his 10th birthday. I then folded the letter and put it in a picture frame behind a photo. Then, to make sure I didn't forget about it, which otherwise would have been close to a 100% possibility, I wrote myself an email reminder for 10 years in the future.

10 years later, I went and found that letter and gave it to him on his 10th birthday. I think it powerfully reinforced the fact that I've climbed a long way to be the guy that stands before him with a multitude of successful companies and loads of employees that call me boss. None of these hold a candle to the amount of love or loyalty I hold for him.... as the only one I get to call son. Here's the letter:

"Hi Noah, I'm your Dad. I'm watching you sleep right now after crying from happiness (I think) for the first time in my life.

Words could never do justice to the crazy array of emotions I'm feeling right now, but I don't know how else or who else to communicate this to, so while these emotions are still fresh, I'm writing a letter for you to open in 10 years.

For starters, I have never been more fucking terrified in my life. I should probably try to stop cussing now that I'm a dad, but I'm 22, which may seem old to you, but is very young to be having a kid especially considering I don't have a penny in the bank, medical insurance, and I'm pretty sure I may have just failed my Junior year of college for missing my marketing final to watch you be born.

I'm going to be WAY more real with you than the average parent is with their kids because I want you to be able to count on what I say... So now may be a good time to tell you I have zero idea what I'm doing or how I'm going to provide for us.

Despite the fact that I have no idea HOW I am going to do it, the HOW somehow seems significantly less important than WHAT you can count on me for, starting right now until the day I die:

1. I'm committed to being a person you can be proud of. I want you to feel a sense of admiration when you tell your friends, "That's my dad." People don't know my name or any of my accomplishments, but just watch; by the time you hear this letter for the second time (or read it yourself at 10 years old), people will have been impacted by what I create and the results of me making this commitment right now.

2. I'm committed to finding a way to produce enough money for you to not just feel secure with the necessities but for you to be able to explore your interests and skills (personally, I am hoping they are Hockey and fighting, but I will support whatever it is as long as you try your ass off at it)...

3. I am now, and will always be, your best friend on the planet. I feel a crazy sense of certainty that I will shift into a whole new realm of stability, productivity, and positivity because that's what needs to happen for me to be the best friend to you, I can be.

For the first time in my life, I want more than I have ever wanted. And ironically, my wanting more has very little to do with ME. It's a weird thing to explain. Hell, it's a weird thing to feel. I don't care if it takes me getting a promotion at the bar or quitting it entirely to figure out and start a business. I don't care if I have to read every single book on parenting, stop partying altogether, finish school in the next year, or drop out and finish later. I won't take a single day off for the next 10 years if that's what it takes to be the type of dad you deserve.

You are 6lbs 6oz of straight-up power and beauty, and I love you with all 162 lbs of me. I have never felt clarity, drive, power, or such a truly deep unconditional love and desire to give.

Look what you have evoked from me, and you aren't even a whole day old yet!

I want everyone to feel what I feel right now, but for the time being, let's just acknowledge that you are a gift. To me and to this planet. I intend on acting like it.

I LOVE YOU WITH EVERYTHING I'VE GOT,

~Your Dad"

Well, it's been a minute since I have read that, and while I sit here with tears in my eyes, I don't know what's more unbelievable... The fact that I was even more syntactically challenged back then or the fact that once upon a time, I only weighed 162 lbs.!

Either way, I think it sets a pretty powerful framework for Noah to look backward and start piling up the endless examples he has witnessed firsthand in his short time here. He can begin connecting the dots from when I was a door-to-door sales guy knocking until my hand was scuffed and bloody while pushing him in a stroller. He can look backward and note the vast percentage of cartoons he watched were at my office with headphones on. He can probably recall climbing on stacks of supplements at the fulfillment center as far back as his memory goes. This is me, putting my money where my mouth is. This is me putting in the hard work to be "the type of dad and friend to him that he deserves" (to quote my highly heartfelt yet poorly handwritten letter).

If I ask him to set the table or put his nose down and push... he knows damn well it's coming from a place I have been myself, attempting to guide him, and our team, to the most desirable destination for both of us.

Final Thoughts On Setting A Good Example:

Finally, I want you to know that while it can be daunting, it is 100% worth seeing our children grow and thrive as people and leaders in their own right. But even more than the joy of being a parent and watching our children become successful, our children give us something equally substantial and profound. The opportunity at the best relationship you've ever had in your life!

Jordan Peterson put it beautifully when he said, "Your kids want to have the best relationship with you they could possibly have. They are 100% on board with that idea. Way more than anybody you have ever met in your life. And that means you could have the best relationship with your children you have ever had with anybody you have ever met, or ever will meet."

Sometimes squeezing an orange can take some effort. But if you are thirsty and vitamin C deprived, to steal a line from the 2004 b list movie "the girl next door" about a dorky kid and a porn star... "The juice is worth the squeeze".

Changing your habits, tonality, or the way you show up in the world to be a better parent is the same. It can, and will be a stretch but believe me when I tell you that with regard to making these changes... the juice is worth the squeeze. And, especially as the behaviors we commit to modeling make our own lives so much more enriched, notwithstanding the added benefit to our beloved offspring. So, let's all agree that we WANT to strive to be the best examples we can be for our kids, one practice and one day at a time.

Chapter 2: Most People Never Listen, Don't Be Most People

(Teaching Communication Skills)

Welcome to Chapter 2. You are about to embark on a journey of discovery, including some uncomfortable truths about communicating, listening, and about your teenager and yourself – but don't worry – it'll soon pass. It will be plain sailing, like a fourth grader taking an astrophysics exam. Kind of. We all want our teenagers to grow up to be successful leaders, at least I know I do, and if you've made it as far as Chapter 2, and that's not what you're looking for, you might want to put this book down and go about your day. There are stores to tend, cities to be built, and AI to hone ready for the end of times. And, if you're Shithead Steve – still reading, sorry, you don't get another mention, so get lost. Now, where was I? Ah yes, teenagers – We want them to have the skills and confidence they need to communicate effectively, inspire others, and achieve their goals. Sounds easy, right? Well, yes and no.

When it comes to developing leadership qualities, communication is key, but let's be honest - talking to teenagers can feel like trying to navigate through a maze blindfolded with one hand tied behind your back. Fret not, avid reader. With the right tools and strategies, all of which you can find in this book (yes, shameless self-promotion alert), we can help our teens become better communicators and leaders. It may take a bit of patience and some serious ninja-level communication skills (I like the way that sounds, but are ninjas even known for their communication skills?), but trust me when I say, it's worth it. Or, as a wise man once said, "The juice is worth the squeeze." Who knows, maybe one day, they'll even be able to have an entire conversation without rolling their eyes or mumbling monosyllabic responses.

How you do anything is how you do everything. Now, you may have heard this quote before, and when I initially heard it, I was kind of skeptical. But think about it. It suggests that how you manage most situations, challenges, or other experiences in your life is probably a good indication of how you handle almost all of the occurrences in your life. Do you ever wonder why you make certain choices? Why you do what you do? Why you like certain things? And why you use the vernacular you use – and how effective it is?

A good question to ask is, what do you want out of life?

A great question to ask is, what pain do you want in your life? What are you willing to struggle for?

Everybody wants an amazing well-paid job, a fantastic relationship, and to be the kind of person that people notice and gravitate to when they walk in the room. Not everyone is willing to struggle through 60-hour work weeks or have the tough conversations to navigate the vulnerability and feelings to cultivate a thriving, vibrant relationship. Many people don't consider the work, effort, and struggle to become a good communicator. Let's take a deeper look at that last one my friends, as that's why we're here - to dive deep into the unknown, the unexplored, and see how really f**ked up you are... I'm kidding, that's why you go to therapy. But... we do want to find what makes you uncomfortable and maybe even consider why? And how we turn that into your superpower (more on superpowers later).

The Importance Of Communication In Leadership

Lincoln, Mandela, and Gandhi – what do they all have in common? Leadership and highly attuned communication skills.

Let's get down to brass tacks: communicating effectively is absolutely crucial if you want to build solid relationships - whether it's with colleagues, neighbors, or your own flesh and blood. Teenagers aren't exactly universally known for their articulate and well-thought-out conversations (unless they're talking about video games or TikTok trends). But teaching your teen how to communicate clearly and authentically will give them a leg up in life. It'll help them gain trust, foster (Noah's middle name) understanding, and achieve common goals with others. And if they've got their sights set on leadership, having killer communication skills is non-negotiable.

When leaders communicate well, they can motivate and inspire others to be their best selves. So don't sleep on this skill - it's a game-changer for your teen's future success.

Let's consider the story of Abraham Lincoln, one of America's greatest leaders, as an example. Aside from arguably some of the strongest facial hair game in history, Lincoln was a master communicator, and he used his skills to inspire his country through some of its most challenging times. His speeches, like the Emancipation Proclamation and the Gettysburg Address, were not only powerful and inspiring but often demonstrated an ability to reach out to his audience and connect with them on an emotional level.

Lincoln was president while the American Civil War was raging. During that time, he gave a speech at a place called Gettysburg. The crux of his address was centered on how important it was that the soldiers who died in battle didn't do so in vain. (No kidding, Abe). He began his speech with the line:

"Four score and seven years ago (his way of saying, "A long, long time ago.") our fathers brought forth on this continent, a new nation, conceived in Liberty, and dedicated to the proposition that all men are created equal."

Lincoln was all about equality and freedom for everyone, and he believed that the Civil War was necessary to ensure that those values would be upheld. He talked about how the soldiers who fought and died at Gettysburg were heroes, and that their sacrifice should inspire us all to keep fighting for what's right, encapsulated in the hugely humble and moving words:

"The world will little note, nor long remember what we say here, but it can never forget what they did here."

He then said, *"It is for us the living, rather, to be dedicated here to the unfinished work which they who fought here have thus far so nobly advanced."*

Ok, history lesson over folks! What's the point? Well, a rough translation of this could be something like: "Hey guys, people died for your future and freedom here - we've got a ton of work to do and a nation to fight for. Time to get to it!" Thanks for the pep talk, Abe. We'll try not to let you down.

Lincoln's speeches have gone down in history because he demonstrated an art and ability to connect with his audience on a personal level. He did this by speaking from the heart and using simple, direct language (Something I am still working on) and was able to inspire his fellow citizens to work together and overcome their differences. He also led by example of the struggle he was willing to endure to fight for what he believed in. That's something as relevant to you, me, and our kids today as at any time in the past.

By communicating effectively, leaders can inspire and motivate others, build strong relationships, and achieve their goals.

Another excellent example of effective communication in leadership is the story of Nelson Mandela, the South African activist who fought against apartheid and became his country's first black president. He brought together people who had been divided by years of racial segregation and inspired them to work together to build a better future. In his famous "I am prepared to die" speech, Mandela concluded by declaring that he had dedicated his whole life to the struggle of black South Africans. Adding that the creation of a free, democratic society, where no race dominates, and all have equal opportunity, was an ideal that he was willing to die for.

Mandela was known for his ability to connect with people from all walks of life and to use humor to break down barriers. During a visit to the United States, Mandela was given a tour of Silicon Valley and was shown the latest computer technology. One of the programmers asked him if he knew how to use a computer.

Mandela replied, "No, but I understand that Bill (Gates) has more money than me, so he can come and teach me."

As you can imagine, this quick wit landed well and made the crowd laugh, putting everyone at complete ease, and even Gates himself found the joke amusing, and it shows Mandela's humility and willingness to learn from others.

As parents, we are the leaders in our teenagers' lives, and it's our responsibility to guide them in learning, practicing, and developing their communication skills. This involves not only teaching them the technical aspects of effective communication, such as speaking clearly and actively listening to others, but also helping them understand the importance of nonverbal communication and how to read social cues. We can model good communication ourselves and spur our teenagers to practice communicating with us and others in a variety of settings. With the right guidance and opportunities, our teenagers can become skilled communicators who are equipped to succeed in all areas of their lives. So how can we teach our teenagers to communicate effectively and become better leaders? Here are my trial-and-error-proven strategies that can help:

Teaching Teenagers Effective Communication Strategies

1. Two Ears, One Mouth: Encourage Active Listening

As Ralph C. Smedley put it, "Real communication is impossible without listening." In fact, Noah and I have a saying in our house that you may steal if you so choose (just make sure you send me my royalty check each time you do…). It goes like this, ready? "LISTENING IS A SUPERPOWER."

We were at a hotel bar while Noah was cutting weight for a tournament in Houston, Texas. With one headphone in and a cowboy hat draped over his face trying to tune out the room, as well as his grumbling stomach and heightened sensitivity to annoying bar chatter.

I shared this saying, "Listening is a superpower," with a fellow day drinker named Carson. He laughed and said, "Ya right, you sound like a self-help author trying to pitch a book on parenting skills." Well, needless to say, his assessment couldn't have been more accurate as the case may now be! But you know what? Even a broken clock is right twice a day… unless it's a broken DIGITAL clock, as they usually do not display time whatsoever, let alone accurately. What was I saying? Oh yea! To prove the accuracy of my aforementioned household slogan, I yelled to a very grumpy hypo-glycemic little weight-cutting Jiu Jitsu powerhouse, "HEY NOAH! What is LISTENING?"

Grumpily, but without hesitation, he yells back in a voice way too loud for the lack of distance between us (hyperbolically mimicking how loud I asked him, clearly), "A SUPERPOWER!". Ahhh, what a fantastic listener he is!

When your teenager learns to listen actively, they will better understand others' perspectives, build stronger relationships, and communicate more effectively. You can encourage your teenager to listen actively to others with verbal cues, like Noah and I, or by paying close attention and trying to investigate the other person, asking open questions, displaying empathy and understanding.

2.   Don't Pick Your Nose in Public: Practice Good Nonverbal Communication

It was Albert Mehrabian, a researcher of body language, who first broke down the components of a face-to-face conversation. He found that communication is 55%

nonverbal, 38% vocal, and 7% words only. Good old Albert, and while those figures and his 55/38/7 formula have been questioned outside of holding a face-to-face conversation with someone as you stare deeply into their wonderful gaze, you might still want to ask yourself how do I sound when I speak? How do I sound when I'm confident? Relaxed? Angry? Or Anxious?

When I started making podcasts for Inside Out Empowerment, I hated hearing my voice, especially when the producer would send me clips to listen back to. Still, the more I listened, the more I understood my voice, its tone, and how I could use that to convey the message I wanted to get across with better impact (thanks, Jacob!). So, one thing you and your teen might want to practice is recording their voice, making podcasts or anything similar they're interested in, and then listening back and trying out different emotions, persuasive arguments, and even role playing selling a product or closing a deal.

So far, I've shared some insight and strategies for developing leadership in your teenager, what a thoroughly wonderous dude I am. But, by hammering home how not to f**k up both your own time on this planet and your young human's, we're going to take a quick look at some things you really ought to avoid. Hopefully, these are already apparent to at least you, otherwise the aforementioned not f**king up your young human may well be beyond the scope of this book, but hey, I love you, and I know you'll make it.

There are many bad nonverbal habits that teenagers and adults can develop. Here are a few examples:

- Avoiding eye contact: When people avoid making eye contact, it can be interpreted as a sign of dishonesty, lack of interest or confidence, or even disrespect.

- Fidgeting: Fidgeting can distract others and make the person doing it seem nervous or unconfident (or like you've had a bag of Colombia's finest export, that stuff will make you fidget like a cat on a hot tin roof).

- Slouching: Poor posture can make a person appear lazy or disinterested. Not forgetting, it can also lead to back problems over time- no one wants to look like a bored Quasimodo when trying to make a good impression.

- Crossed arms: When a person crosses their arms, it can make them appear defensive or closed off, and can also be seen as a sign of disinterest.

- Playing with hair or jewelry: This can be distracting to others and can also make the person doing it appear nervous or unprofessional.

- Interrupting: Interrupting others can be seen as rude and disrespectful and can also make the person doing it appear impatient, arrogant, or unaware. One simple, yet effective strategy is to pause or count to two in your head before replying (Remember, count in your head - or you're gonna come across like a roadie testing a concert stage mic).

- Speaking too quickly or too slowly: Speaking too quickly can make it difficult for others to understand what the person is saying, while speaking too slowly can make the person appear hesitant or unconfident.
- Using filler words: Filler words such as "um," "like," and "you know" can make a person appear unprofessional, unclear, and unprepared.

According to the 55/38/7 formula, nearly 40% of a person's attitude is conveyed vocally through tone and inflection, so try to ensure that your tone matches whatever message you're trying to convey. You can also try speaking in a deeper voice. Research has shown that people who speak with a low-pitched voice are rated more authoritative and competent than those who speak with a higher pitch. A good trick for this, is to practice some diaphragmatic breathing. If you breathe deeply into the bottom of your belly (pushing your naval out as you inhale) prior to speaking, just watch how much richer and full bodied, if not outright deeper, the tone of your voice becomes.

Nonverbal communication is an integral part of effective communication. By highlighting it and practicing it yourself, you can inspire your teenager to practice good nonverbal communication skills, like maintaining eye contact, using appropriate gestures (and not picking their nose in public), and using a clear and confident tone of voice. These skills can help project confidence and build trust in others.

Still, to this day, the most quintessential example of somebody I've watched masterfully displaying powerful non-verbal communication was some guy named Tony. Tony Robbins 😊.

I was 19 years old, and my awesome aunt Bonnie hooked my brother Ben and me up with tickets to his Unleash the Power Within seminar. Reticent as I was, I really looked up to Bonnie, so I agreed, packed my bags, and headed to Colorado Springs, CO.

While the content of the seminar was very engaging, insightful, fun, and uplifting, I was fixated on how incredible of a presence Tony had. Almost at will, he seemed to jerk a crowd of 10,000 from one emotional state to another.

I had to figure out how he was doing it, so I started researching the guy. As it turns out, he was not just born this behemoth-sized master of communication. He had a lot of help from his training in something called Neuro-Linguistic Programming.

NLP (Neuro-Linguistic Programming) is described as a pseudoscientific approach to communication, personal development, and psychotherapy. It was introduced in Richard Bandler and John Grinder's 1975 book "The Structure of Magic I." NLP suggests that there is a connection between neurological processes, language, and acquired behavioral patterns, and that these connections can be modified to achieve specific life goals. Bandler and Grinder assert that NLP has the potential to address various issues such as phobias, depression, tic disorders, psychosomatic illnesses, near-sightedness, allergies, the common cold, and learning disorders, often claiming effectiveness in just one session. Additionally, they propose that NLP can be used to model the skills of exceptional individuals, enabling anyone to acquire those skills.

I looked up the closest school that taught NLP, and in the true addict brain obsessively minded way I approach many things, decided to get my basic certification. This process had me drilling techniques and learning principles 10-12 hours per day for about two weeks. While I did not become Tony Robbins, it did give me some solid foundational concepts and practices I've been able to draw on in many circumstances over the years, and I believe they are helpful enough to pass to you here.

NLP is most commonly known for its use by pickup artists. While I'm sure your teen may appreciate, and even thank you for this kind of insight – we'll be looking at NLP in an entirely different way. Let's start by looking at "Mirroring", which refers to the practice of reflecting or mirroring a person's language and communication style in order to build rapport and establish trust. In short, using similar language, tone, and pace as the person you are communicating with to create a sense of connection and understanding without overdoing it and coming off as a weirdo. It is often used by therapists, coaches, and salespeople to build rapport with clients or customers. It may sound odd that simply by somebody holding the same physical body posture as you or slightly adopting your vocal intonation, will make you like them more, but the subconscious sense of familiarity is a real phenomenon. Try it!

Positive body language; think long hair, head down, earbuds in… ok maybe not. But body language is another rapport-building technique that can be particularly effective for teenagers, chiefly because they often struggle with positive body language at this stage of life. A genuine smile can convey warmth and friendliness and can help to put the other person at ease. Gentle eye contact shows that you're paying attention and are engaged in the conversation. (Obviously, no one wants to get into an awkward accidental starring contest, so you might want to point that out from the start).

Another way to do this is by facing the person you're speaking to rather than turning away or looking elsewhere. This shows that you're focused on them and interested in what they have to say. Instead, it's much better to keep your body open and relaxed, with your arms at your sides, and my notes say, "or resting on a table," which obviously requires a table in your vicinity, or you'll go to lean and end up on the floor looking embarrassed, and less than open to communicating. See folks, all the best tips throughout this book. I'm thinking about that shiny review you're going to leave me. Ah ha! This book writing game, pfft, nothing to it! (*wipes sweat from brow).

3. Gimme Your Best Dad Joke: Use Humor to Break the Ice

Humor can transform a dull and dreary conversation into a lively and engaging one just as easily as it can deescalate a situation if people are becoming too tense or heated. The first situation that jumped out at me demonstrating this was when we were negotiating the purchase of a property out in Las Vegas that wasn't going very well. As a heated argument broke out amongst the executives, my dad waited for about 10 minutes before jumping in with a classic tension breaker: "So, gentlemen, how's your sex life?" The ill-timed (or brilliantly timed, depending on the viewpoint) comment, combined with his nonchalantness, paralyzed the argument for a moment. Everyone stopped and paused to process what he'd said and then fell into fits of laughter, and the tension vanished into thin air.

Another example of the Ice or Tension being broken with humor I can think of is during the whole Bill Clinton and Monica Lewinsky scandal. He was about to go on air and be publicly raked over the coals for his indiscretions, and the tension in the room apparently reflected it.

JFK Jr., with impeccable timing, faxed directly into the oval office a picture of himself at probably 5 or 6 under the desk while his father, JFK Sr., was on a phone call (an iconic image from his father's presidency) along with the caption "If I could barely fit under there as a small child, I have a hard time envisioning an intern doing so." Needless to say, it made the room burst out laughing and created an ally out of the administration that would later go on to support him in a magazine endeavor surrounding pop culture and politics.

Now, I know what you're thinking - how can this help with communicating with teenagers? Well, friends, let me tell you that teenagers can be a tough nut to crack when it comes to communication. They may be reluctant to talk or only respond with a grunt or a monosyllabic word. But humor can be your secret weapon to break through their tough exterior. You can tell them a joke, share a funny story, or even just use a playful tone of voice while asking a serious question. This can help to lighten the mood and embolden your teenager to open up, share their thoughts, and in turn, develop their own unique communication style. So, never underestimate the power of humor in communication, especially when it comes to teenagers.

4. To Be, Or Not To Be: Use Role-Playing Exercises

Oh, role-playing exercises, now that sounds like a lot of fun, doesn't it? I mean, who doesn't love pretending to be someone else for a little while? It's like Halloween every day, except without the candy, the scary costumes, or the spooky decorations. Okay, maybe it's not exactly like Halloween, but it's still pretty cool. And you know what makes it even cooler? Using it to help your teenager practice their communication skills.

Role-playing exercises allow you to explore, take on different roles and act out real-world scenarios from that role's perspective. You could practice handling conflict, making a persuasive argument, or even arguing for something you don't actually believe in. Maybe you could argue that pineapple pizza is the best pizza, even though you secretly hate it (sorry, pineapple pizza lovers. For the record, I am one of your kind).

But here's the thing, these exercises aren't just fun and games, they're also super effective. By practicing these scenarios in a safe, controlled environment, your teenager can build their confidence, improve their communication skills, and learn how to handle difficult situations with ease. So, why not give it a try? Who knows, you might even discover your hidden talent for improv! Here are a few more ideas for you to consider:

- Practice communication: Role-playing allows teenagers to practice their communication skills in a safe and supportive environment. They can experiment with different ways of expressing themselves and receive feedback on how they come across to others.

- Handling conflict: Conflict resolution is an important skill for leaders, and role-playing can help teenagers practice how to handle difficult conversations or disputes. They can practice active listening, expressing themselves assertively and respectfully, and finding common ground with others.

- Persuasion: Role-playing can help teenagers practice making persuasive arguments, which is a critical leadership skill. They can practice presenting their ideas in a clear and compelling way, anticipating objections, and addressing them effectively.

- Empathy: We'll touch on empathy fully in Chapter 7, but for now keep in mind that role-playing can also help teenagers develop empathy, because as they play different roles, they are simultaneously and inadvertently putting into practice placing themselves in others' shoes, emotions and perspectives. Let's dig a little deeper, it's our job to teach our teens, as well as ourselves, the value in releasing our innate self-centeredness, and to start seeing things from other people's perspectives! This means developing emotional intelligence and becoming more empathetic. Let's be honest, we could all use a bit more of that in the world. What can that look like in action? Well, I once witnessed a class on empathy at Noah's school. Imagine having that topic to teach a bunch of teenagers and keep them interested! But the teacher was astute and had a trick up her sleeve – a game with blindfolds and verbal cues, that involved teamwork with pairs of students guiding each other to navigate around the classroom. The first pair, let's call them Mike and Emily, were doing pretty well until Mike tripped and fell. And what did he say? "That's the last time I take directions from a girl!" The whole class started laughing, while the teacher used it as an opportunity to get the kids talking about the importance of understanding someone else's perspective and viewing the world through their eyes as a demonstration of how empathy works. Brilliant! Meanwhile, Mike never walked again... Ok, I made that part up. To clarify, Mike was fine, and no Mike's were harmed in the telling of this story. Despite what my dramatic side suggests.

5. Fetch My Megaphone: Provide Opportunities for Public Speaking

Public speaking isn't just for politicians and motivational speakers, it's a crucial skill for effective leadership. And lucky for us, our teenagers can start developing this skill right now! We just need to give them a little push and encouragement.

Think about it - the ability to communicate effectively in front of a crowd is priceless. Whether it's impressing the fam at Thanksgiving dinner or wowing the audience at the school talent show, our teens can shine like the stars they are. And let's not forget about the real-world applications of public speaking. Job interviews, presentations, and even everyday conversations with colleagues can all benefit from this skill.

So, how do we get our teens on board? Easy. We can fire them up to join a public speaking club or participate in public speaking opportunities whenever they can. It could be as simple as asking them to talk at a family gathering or present a talk at a school event. And the best part? This not only builds their confidence but also hones their communication skills and also helps them develop their leadership potential. Not to mention learning to deal with the internal battle that arises as the emotions swirl and adrenaline starts to grip them prior to standing up.

Every year, Noah used to make it a personal goal to be the highest earner at his elementary school's yearly fundraiser called "The Fun Run". Parents (and maybe the occasional neighbor or two) would contribute to students by pledging to donate a minimum of $1 for each lap the student could run within a specific time frame. Students would then be rewarded for the amount they raised per lap.

The vast majority of prizes were nominal at best and ranged everything from a beach ball at $1 per lap, to a pathetic excuse for a bracelet that hugged your wrist when you slapped it. (I'm not saying slap bracelets weren't fantastic, but if you raised $12 bucks per lap and you ended up running 50 laps... do the math.) Whoever set up this prize structure was either a genius or really needed to step up his game in the compensation department, not totally sure which.

The absolute grand prize was, however, pretty cool each year. Although most of them are slipping my mind at the moment. I think the last year of elementary school, at $50 per lap, was an Oculus virtual reality gaming system. However, by this time, Noah had done these enough years in a row for both of us to know that the "Grand Prize" was simply Noah's starting point.

While most kids were embarking on their obtain-the-gaming-console mission, during which they would burn out and get discouraged or distracted, falling far short of the necessary funds raised, Noah was setting out to ensure nobody (no matter how high they climbed the ladder) would be able to match his dollar contribution.

In the last year of Noah's elementary school career, I believe he raised almost double the amount necessary to take home the grand prize. At $97 per lap raised with maximum laps run capped at 36 laps (a very physically achievable goal given the allotted amount of time), Noah raised just shy of $3,600 himself for the school and a charity for underprivileged children. This apparently was not only the highest quantity raised by a student that year, but the highest quantity raised by a student, ever.

After the fun run each year was a ceremony where the kids got to see their cumulative contribution to a good cause and, of course, their individual prizes. Before the assembly, the coordinator of the fun run "Captain Craig" (not entirely sure that was his legal name as I didn't check his license, but then again, I didn't know I would one day, many years later, be writing this book) pulled us aside along with the principle and said we don't have any additional prizes above $50 per lap and you did almost double. What can we do to reward you or acknowledge the additional contribution?

An idea popped into my head, I pulled Noah aside and said, "Hey buddy, while we have everyone gathered here... how would you feel about talking to them about how you did it?"

He wasn't opposed to the idea but asked what he would say. We requested 10 minutes so he and I could discuss, and we made a list of all the things he did. Walking around my office pitching employees on the value of how the money would be spent and asking for donations, making a list of every single person he knew or could think of that he could make a phone call to, making a list of friends and family members of other students that they didn't want to call, etc. All of which were things he did, by the way.

Partway through the brainstorming session, he said, "OK, stop Dad, I have enough!" Sure as shit, the little bugger walks back up to the guy and says, "OK, I'm ready. When it's my turn, call me up or come get me. I'm in Mrs. Morrison's class." then goes back to his spot at the assembly.

He gets called to the stage and straight-up crushes it. Not because he'd be graded an A from the local chapter of Toastmasters with a rubric in front of them but because he manned (or womaned) up and spoke from the heart. His friggin' adorable speech intro went something like this:

"I have always tried really hard at this fundraiser, and because of that, I do really good at it. This year I did good enough that they are letting me talk to you about it because that's what I asked for. After all... if you don't ask, you don't get. My dad told me that because his dad told him that, and now I'm telling you that because if all of us tried as hard as we could and did the right things.... we could raise way more money for good causes, and all get way better prizes. So basically, here's what I did..."

I don't think up until that point I had ever been prouder of him in my life. His speech ended, and somehow the audience reciprocated the fact that if they listened to him, they would all get better rewards AND make a bigger difference. It finished with the crowd cheering, "NOAH! NOAH! NOAH!" and he quite literally dropped the mic.

As he exited, I gave him our father-son handshake and asked him how stoked he was about how that just went. He replied, "I'm sorry to cuss, but that was the scariest fuckin' thing I've ever done in my life and I'm so glad it's over."

I asked, "Are you happy you did it?"

He goes, "Duh Dad, were you even listening?"

Aside from the fact that I don't think I've ever been so proud in my entire life prior to his athletic career starting, it brought me face to face with the fact that every time we overcome ourselves, we love ourselves a little more…

What better excuse to do precisely that than speaking in front of a crowd where you are ALSO forced to organize your thoughts in a cohesive trackable way and remain composed and coherent while your emotions are running wild?

6.   Put the Baseball Bat Down: Practice Nonviolent Communication

Nonviolent Communication (NVC) is a method of communication that was created by psychologist Marshall Rosenberg. It is centered around expressing ourselves in a way that is both truthful and respectful while avoiding any threat of harm to the other person. The process involves recognizing and articulating our own feelings and needs, clearly and honestly, without resorting to blame or criticism towards others. It also emphasizes the importance of compassion, empathy, and understanding as the foundation for successful communication.

The main objective of NVC is to promote connection and cooperation instead of conflict and defensiveness. Through this approach, individuals can better understand one another and work towards mutually beneficial solutions. NVC is applicable in various settings, whether it is in personal relationships, workplace interactions, or community engagement. By adopting NVC principles, individuals can build stronger and more harmonious relationships. Covering more ground, without the wasted energy of an avoidable conflict.

Here are some techniques that can be used in Nonviolent Communication:

- Observation: Start by observing and describing the situation objectively, without judgment or evaluation. For example, "When I saw you didn't clean the dishes, I felt frustrated."
- Feeling: Express your feelings about the situation, using "I" statements. For example, "I feel frustrated when I see the dishes not being cleaned."
- Need: Identify the underlying need or value that is driving your feelings. For example, "I have a need for cleanliness and order in our shared living space."

- Request: Make a clear, specific request for what you want the other person to do. For example, "Would you be willing to clean the dishes now, or at least let me know when you plan to do it?"

If you wanna avoid punching each other in the face and actually communicate with your teenager, you should try nonviolent communication. It's like a cheat code that helps you both express your feelings and needs without resorting to throwing punches or insults. While your language does not necessarily need to be as robotic as in the examples above, trust me when I tell you that this framework is like a Jedi mind trick for communication. And let's be real, who doesn't want to be a Jedi? So, give it a try, and may the force be with you.

Through NVC, you can cultivate a greater sense of understanding and cooperation, which can help reduce conflicts and bring about solution-oriented collaboration. Hell, if you get good enough at it, the added rapport may even deepen the connectivity of the bond! Honing your capacity for NVC is especially crucial for effective leadership, where leaders must often navigate complex and challenging situations diligently and seamlessly.

By practicing NVC together, you'll create a family environment so harmonious and connected that even your great aunt Mavis will stop nagging you about when you're having another kid. Plus, your teenager will be set up for success as a compassionate and effective leader - you know, the kind of person who gets stuff done without being a total ass about it. You and your teen can communicate your needs and desires in a way that's respectful, compassionate, and non-judgmental - which is especially useful when you're trying to avoid a fight with a family member about whose turn it is to do the dishes. So, teach your teen how to communicate like a pro, and watch them blossom into a master of diplomacy, tact, and effectiveness

7. Don't be a Pleb: Promote Reading, Writing & Journaling

Effective communication isn't just about yapping away or listening attentively. It's about the whole shebang - reading, writing, and maybe even telepathy if you're into that sort of thing. Reading helps expand our vocabulary and introduces us to new ideas, like how to train a dragon or the importance of always carrying a towel. If those two aren't your bag, I know a guy that writes a few grand slam how-to books on productivity and overcoming overthinking (cough, check out my Author Page on Amazon, cough). Meanwhile, writing is like a mental gym that helps us flex our brain muscles and organize our thoughts. And let's be honest, who doesn't love a smooth flowing expression that expands the mind or shifts our position?

These skills are particularly crucial for our teenagers, who are about to face the world of higher education and the workforce. In these arenas, being able to communicate in a cogent and logical manner is the difference between success and ending up living in your parents' basement until you're 40. We should rally our teens to read, write, and think critically, because that's how we raise the next generation of witty, charming, and persuasive communicators.

Let's be honest here, teens by-in-large have a lot of pent-up emotions that can make them feel like they're about to explode at any moment. But fear not, my friend, because regular journaling can help them make sense of all those feelings and even prevent any potential emotional outbursts. It's like a therapist but way cheaper. Not only that, but journaling can also unleash their inner creative genius and improve their writing skills. Who knows, maybe your kid will be the next J.K. Rowling. Or, you know, just end up a slightly better communicator… both are wins if you ask me.

Incorporating reading and writing into our teenagers' daily routines can also have long-term benefits for their academic and professional success. Strong reading and writing skills are essential for success in many fields, and by developing these skills at a young age, our teenagers will have a strong foundation for their future endeavors.

- Here are a few ideas broken down:
- Self-reflection: Journaling can help teenagers develop self-awareness by encouraging them to reflect on their thoughts, feelings, and experiences. This can help them better understand their own motivations, values, and beliefs.
- Emotional regulation: Writing down emotions can help teenagers process and regulate their feelings. By identifying and acknowledging their emotions,

teenagers can better manage their reactions to stressful or difficult situations.

- Creativity: Journaling can be a creative outlet for teenagers, allowing them to express themselves through writing, drawing, or other artistic means. This can help them explore their own interests and passions and develop their creative skills.

- Goal setting: By keeping track of their progress towards personal goals, teenagers can develop a sense of accomplishment and motivation to continue working towards their aspirations. We take a deeper look at goal setting in Chapter 6, so you can jump forward and take a look, or just know that now is a great time to get them into the habit of writing.

- Prompt Responses: Taking a moment to consider and reflect upon a question for a few moments. While it is beneficial to exercise the muscle, it's also helpful to get outside of ourselves for a moment when our thoughts are too loud. When in doubt, focus out!

I highly recommend journaling as a means of self-improvement. The ancient philosopher Epictetus was all about it, and he was a pretty wise dude. He galvanized his students to keep a journal to reflect on their actions and progress toward their goals. It's called "The View from Above," which sounds like some kind of mystical, transcendental experience, but really, it's just imagining yourself rising above your current situation to gain a broader perspective on your life and circumstances. No big deal, right?

The Stoics were profound journalers, and their style of journaling involves reflecting on your actions, thoughts, and emotions, and analyzing them from a rational and objective perspective. Basically, you're looking at yourself like a scientist studying a lab rat. But in a good way. By examining your own behavior and reactions to events, you can develop greater self-awareness and emotional regulation, and identify areas for self-improvement.Consider encouraging your teen to start journaling. It's a valuable tool for their personal growth and self-improvement. Plus, they'll get to explore their creative side and improve their writing skills. Who knows, maybe they'll even become the next great Stoic philosopher.

Mastering The Art Of Effective Communication: An Invaluable Skill For All

If you want to really nail this communication thing, there are a few key takeaways you need to remember. First off, empathy and active listening are key. Secondly, give your teens the opportunity to speak in public or in front of a group to hone their skills. Thirdly, practice nonviolent communication and avoid throwing blame around. Fourthly, encourage reading, writing, and journaling to improve vocabulary and critical thinking skills. And finally, remember that this is a process that requires patience and consistency. With a little effort, we can help our teenagers become the best versions of themselves and unleash their full potential as leaders.

I think I wrote these Final Thoughts while overtired, and upon second reflection feel as though it bears a striking resemblance to a conclusion paragraph to one of my high school sophomore year essays that was primarily derived from a spark notes depiction of "A Tale of Two Cities". Syntactically correct with very little heart or intellectual assimilation of any of the aforementioned principles.

Let's back it up for a second. Put yourself in the shoes of the listener, be it a massive audience during a public speech or your singular child. What makes you want to express yourself fully? I'd venture to guess, a person (or persons) that WANT to hear you out, and who indicate their understanding as you speak, probably doesn't hurt your willingness or ability to expound upon your position. Emulate those traits while you're being communicated with.

When you've done such an incredible job being an audience for your kids that they've developed an aptitude for expressing themselves, get creative in order for them to do the same in front of an audience that is larger than just you! Preferably do this more than once or twice, as speaking publicly will become a second nature element to organizing their thoughts in a comprehensible manner. Doing so proficiently will only contribute to their competence and confidence as a young leader.

When they attempt to do any of these things and run into the normal frustration they will assuredly face, giving them tools to deal with it besides casting aspersions and throwing temper tantrums is not just ideal, but entirely necessary. The higher they aim, the more frustration and reward are guaranteed to accompany the process. If they want the prize, it's imperative they have pragmatic skills and strategies to reach their lofty aims.

Lastly, find books they like reading. If they suck at reading, you can practice, sure, but you can also use audible so they can try using their ears instead of deciphering words. Find prompts they like writing and responding to. If they have the writing of an autistic preschooler (which once upon a time I DID because once upon a time I WAS), use voice to text or some other means of expressing their thoughts that doesn't require them being caught up on the element that shines a light on their shortcomings.

If we create an environment that plays to their strengths, our kids, like any humans, will lean into understanding. They will lean into expression. They will lean into all the awesome things that we humans do innately prior to attempting to shove ourselves into a box that doesn't fit our natural form of communication in one way or another.

If, as a parent, you have the capacity to gently yet powerfully step out of the way of normalcy in order to easily create said environment, just watch as your future leader effortlessly enjoys flexing the necessary skills over and over again until he or she seemingly innately develops the communication capacity of a natural born leader.

Chapter 3: Analyze Strengths and Weaknesses

In the grand scheme of things, it's damn helpful for folks to recognize their abilities early on. Supporting your teen to get a grip on their strengths and weaknesses from the get-go lets them zero in on honing those strengths and unleashing the skills that come naturally to them.

As our teens dig deep and do some self-analysis, they'll uncover their kickass qualities and the areas where they need a little extra attention, all in the pursuit of building a strong, well-rounded personality. As parents, educators, or mentors, we hold the privilege of helping our teenagers nurture self-awareness and grasp the intricacies of their distinctive strengths and weaknesses.

When we guide our teenagers to reflect on their abilities, values, and passions, we empower them to embark on a journey of self-awareness that will shape their leadership, and without being grandiose, life trajectory.

This is a topic that I've spoken passionately about in the past, on the Inside Out Empowerment Podcast (hosted by some guy named Joshua Nussbaum, you may have heard of him), Episode 4 – Strengthening Self Confidence Through Self Validation. I want to share with you a short exert from that episode, which very nearly went into Chapter 5 on Building Confidence, and there is some overlap, but I think the importance of this dialogue fits just as well, if not better here, and it's my book, so here's the exert:

"In today's session were going to be discussing the concept and very important muscle of self validation. Self validation is something that I know I had to develop, acknowledging and recognizing my own strengths, and reinforcing them when I do a good job.

It's something that I've seen amongst many other leaders of large organizations, teams, and successful athletes, have the capacity to recognize the things that they do well. The definition of validation is recognition or affirmation that a person or their feelings and opinions are valid or worthwhile. If you ever want to be a mover or shaker and create something of value and have the courage to travel your own path, you have to have the ability to look internally and acknowledge what is, and acknowledge your weaknesses openly and honestly with yourself. Develop a capacity to be able to recognize your strengths and your positive actions.

Self validation is a really ironic dichotomy because people confuse it with ego, and it really is not ego. In fact, ironically most of the people with a very large ego externally, are that way because they have an inability to flow hardcore self-love, so they develop a hard exterior, showing the world that they are unaffected and that they don't need your approval or your support. Ironically, the people that can really acknowledge the things that they're super good at as well as the things that they're not so good at are generally more raw, vulnerable, and honest.

When you're communicating with them, they're more capable of receiving feedback. So, one of the things I'm inviting you to do through today's session is, drop the guard a little bit, drop whatever predisposition or prejudice you have about telling yourself that you're fucking awesome, and being able to take a hard look at yourself and communicate to yourself internally. What it is that you enjoy about yourself. You know I developed a practice throughout a really awesome leadership seminar that I did, where they forced us to write love letters to ourselves on a daily basis.

It's a practice that seemed really goofy at first, but that's what's actually inspiring today's topic, as I recently stumbled across an old journal from 2014, years ago, and I wasn't quite as established. I was in a little bit of a difficult position financially, but emotionally incredibly strong, and writing to myself frequently. I stumbled across one of these letters which inspired me to talk about the purpose of being able to hold your position in space. Being able to be unshakeable, and that starts with a foundation of being able to acknowledge what it is that you're good at.

I'm inviting you to drop the necessity to externally defend yourself, your beliefs, your positions, or your actions, because in reality that generally derives from a position of feeling insecure. Internally all of us are most certainly the hardest critics. So instead of being externally brash, harsh, and defensive, then internally, being overly critical...I would like to invite you to practice internally being incredibly loving, and then just watch what happens externally as a result.

One of my favorite quotes that T. Harv Eker said, or wrote I should say, in "Secrets of the Millionaire Mind" which is a great book for up-and-coming budding entrepreneurs, is 'whatever you put your attention on, expands.' It might sound silly to sit there and say, "Hey, I really loved the way you brushed your teeth this morning, got out of bed, set your kid up for success, cooked him an awesome breakfast, reinforced the fact that he's an awesome bad ass, you know is in control of his environment. I sent him to school with a kiss, and a hug, and some positivity, so that he could be the best 3rd grader he could possibly be, and then you went to the office. You really gave it your best! I really liked the way you handled your phone call with so and so" but you know, what you put your attention on expands. If at the end of the day you don't have the ability to say, "Hey, atta boy Joshua" if your name's Joshua (that's what I say!), you're going to need to start searching for it externally. So, operating from the position of what you put your attention on expands, as you continue to validate yourself for the things that you're doing well in life, you're going to notice a beautiful phenomenon occur; that those pieces you do well start to become a dominate force in your personality!

It's not that you ignore your shortcomings, or that you're not constantly working on yourself. But by developing the muscle, which is all it really is, to say hey, I did these three things really frickin' well today, and I want to acknowledge you, or acknowledge myself for xyz, it programmes your subconscious mind to a) Say that you're doing something well – which builds self-confidence and reassures your position in the world. b) It's going to strengthen those qualities within yourself.

You know, in such a socially connected world, I've noticed that we've started to rely on external validation as a reinforcement way too much. Self-validation strengthens our core and internal confidence, giving us the capacity to create and to develop, to adventure and to be a pioneer, in spite of the nay-sayers. You know, truth is not determined by a majority vote, so don't f**king act like it is. I really love that quote because so many people have an idea, or a concept, or are enthused about something, and then, they allow their bubble to be popped because they share it with someone else before it's a proven concept, and then they haven't enrolled other people in their vision yet. If you wanna have the capacity to develop that ability to feel good and build security where you're an unshakable force you've got to develop the capacity to develop and acknowledge what it is that you do well."

So, with all that said - Let this chapter be a roadmap for helping your kid navigate the terrain of self-discovery. As we traverse practical steps like self-reflection, seeking feedback, conducting assessments, and setting goals. By following these steps, your teenager will gain clarity about their abilities, areas for improvement, and personal aspirations.

Cracking The Leadership Code: Analyzing Strengths And Weaknesses

"Leadership is not just about charisma and personality. It's about taking responsibility, practicing discipline, and making the right decisions, even when they are difficult."

– Jim Collins

Self-awareness is a fundamental aspect of effective leadership. Let's be real, we've probably all experienced or seen leaders in various walks of life, from work to government who don't fully exhibit the self-awareness trait, and it's often painful, to say the least.

Leaders who understand their strengths can use them to inspire and motivate others. Meanwhile, those who recognize their weaknesses can work on improving and surround themselves with complementary team members. By analyzing strengths and weaknesses, teenagers can make informed choices, set realistic goals, and cultivate the skills necessary for well-rounded leadership.

Leadership is an ongoing journey of growth and learning and one element of this journey is identifying and developing your strengths to make sound decisions for your team. It takes a strong leader to bring out the best in their employees (especially the difficult or lazy ones!), drive innovation and get everyone on the same page pulling in the same direction. Conversely, self-aware leaders who understand their limitations and work on them or use effective delegation are more relatable, trustworthy and authentic.

At its core, leadership is about influencing and motivating others to achieve a shared goal. It entails setting a vision and mobilizing people to work together toward that vision. There are a number of leadership styles, and various methods leader use to motivate and encourage their teams to achieve goals. but for brevity, let's take a quick glance at the four main types:

1. Authoritarian Leadership: An authoritarian leader is characterized by a strong emphasis on control and decision-making power. They typically make decisions independently and expect strict adherence to their instructions. This style can be effective in situations that require quick decision-making or in environments where clear hierarchies are necessary. However, it may hinder creativity and employee empowerment.

2. Democratic Leadership: Democratic leaders value input and participation from their team members. They encourage open communication, collaboration, and shared decision-making. This style fosters a sense of inclusivity and empowers employees by involving

them in the decision-making process. It can enhance morale, creativity, and innovation within the team.

3. Transformational Leadership: Transformational leaders inspire and motivate their teams to achieve exceptional performance. They exhibit charismatic qualities and provide a compelling vision for the future. These leaders focus on personal growth, development, and mentoring. They encourage their team members to reach their full potential and create a positive work environment. Transformational leadership can lead to high levels of employee engagement and loyalty.

4. Transactional Leadership: Transactional leaders focus on setting clear expectations and providing rewards or punishments based on performance. They establish specific goals and reward employees when those goals are met. Transactional leaders emphasize structure, rules, and accountability. While this style can ensure compliance and efficiency, it may not foster creativity or intrinsic motivation.

The most effective leaders are adaptable, adjusting their style to fit each situation. A leader might excel in delegating tasks but struggle with public speaking. This self-awareness empowers leaders to develop their skillset and build a well-rounded leadership style that can adapt to different situations and better meet their team's needs, and it all flows from analyzing strengths and weaknesses.

The Power Of Self-Reflection And Guiding Your Teen In Analyzing Strengths And Weaknesses

Analyzing strengths and weaknesses can be massive for our teenager's development. It enables them to confidently leverage their strengths, build self-awareness, enhance decision-making, and embrace opportunities for growth. By sitting down and dedicating some time and effort to this process, our teens can find ways to optimize their potential, ignite their own inspiration (and in others), and effectuate a meaningful and far-reaching impact within their peer groups, teams, communities and beyond.

And I want to give a quick mention here to attributes. Well, I hear you ask, what about attributes? Attributes are those innate qualities that shape our identity, are deeply ingrained within us. From the moment we enter the world, we possess varying degrees of each Attribute, which define our strengths, weaknesses, and how we navigate diverse circumstances.

It's easy to succumb to the misconception that there exists a fixed and "correct" set of Attributes, but this notion is far from reality. Different Attributes prove advantageous in different situations. What truly matters is having the Attributes required to tackle the specific tasks at hand.

But what lies at the heart of this phenomenon? What scientific explanations underlie the connection between Attributes and individuality? Surely, there must be reasons why specific Attributes shape someone's character and why each person possesses a distinct combination of them. Well, I invite you to check out www.theattributes.com where they've developed three distinct self-assessment tools that measure Grit, Mental Acuity and Drive.

Setting the stage for understanding and assessing strengths and weaknesses

Adolescence can be a rollercoaster of emotions, so we want our teens to feel safe to explore their strengths and weaknesses without fear of judgment. This way, they'll feel comfortable being honest and open about their abilities and limitations. It'll do wonders for their self-esteem.

Here are some wider points to consider:

- Self-awareness and personal growth: Taking a good, hard look at our strengths and weaknesses can be like finding out that you can do a flawless backflip but struggle to open a pickle jar. By uncovering their quirks, talents, and areas with room for improvement, our teenagers can laser-focus their efforts on honing their skills.
- Maximizing strengths: When teenagers are aware of their strengths, they can leverage them to bring out the best in themselves and those around them. By capitalizing on their natural abilities and talents, they can inspire, motivate, and influence others. Understanding their strengths allows teenagers to take on leadership roles that align with their unique skill sets, increasing their chances of success and

fulfillment. To that end here are some questions you can ask you teenager or nudge them toward reflecting on:

a) What are my passions and hobbies? Do I like these activities because of certain skills I possess?

b) What do others say I am good at?

c) What kind of tasks am I able to do quickly?

d) Which activities take me longer? Which skills are important for these tasks?

e) In which tasks do I require assistance?

- Addressing weaknesses: By analyzing their not-so-superhero powers, teenagers can unleash their inner training montage and proactively work on developing the skills they need to overcome limitations. This whole process cultivates a growth mindset where weaknesses are seen as opportunities for growth, not as permanent blemishes and start the process of transforming themselves into the most well-rounded leaders the world has ever seen. Who said superheroes couldn't have a few quirks, right?

- Effective decision-making: With a crystal-clear understanding of their strengths, teenagers can make choices that match the areas they enjoy, where they have expertise and passion. By acknowledging their weaknesses, they gain insight into their current limitations and can make smart decisions. From there, they can seek guidance from others who excel in those areas, collaborate, or even come up with clever strategies to outsmart any potential limitations. Understanding their strengths and weaknesses is a hugely enlightening and important field in self-growth, building leadership skills and crucially, at least for this point, making effective decisions, so much so, that the next chapter is dedicated to just that, making decisions (see what I did there!).

When we think about self-reflection, we're not talking about gazing into a mirror and asking deep existential questions (although that could be fun too).

As mentors, parents, or educators, it's our chance to offer some well-meaning, constructive feedback. But let's remember, we're not here to crush dreams or rain on parades. It's all about helping them understand themselves better.

Be supportive and provide specific and actionable feedback. Highlight their strengths, those moments when they shine, and gently point out areas where they can grow and improve. Introduce them to self-assessment tools and guide them through the process, then help them interpret the results. One such resource is the Free Aptitude Test for Strengths and Weaknesses found at www.richardstep.com, the test takes 10-12 minutes and promises to give you your top 5 strengths and your bottom weakness.

Suddenly, your teen will have a structured framework to objectively assess their abilities and preferences. This can be a light bulb moment for our kids when everything starts to make sense.

By establishing a foundation for comprehending and evaluating strengths and weaknesses, we equip our prospective leaders with the necessary tools to navigate their voyage of self-discovery, they'll gain valuable insights into their abilities and passions, and with this new self-awareness be guided toward their full leadership potential and making a meaningful impact in their lives and the world around them.

Here are a few areas to practice with your teen:

- Seeking feedback: Inspire your teenager to seek advice from mentors, peers, and teachers. We want to create a culture where open communication and constructive criticism are normalized, and seen as a platform for awareness and growth.

- Conducting assessments: We're talking personality tests, SWAT skills inventories, and more. These assessments help them see their natural talents and areas where they could use a little work, a bit like having a cheat code to unlock the secrets of their unique abilities.

- Recognizing patterns: challenge your teenager to be like Sherlock Holmes and look for recurring patterns and behaviors. Do they excel in certain situations? Do they trip over the same hurdles every time? Spotting these patterns allows them to determine their strengths, weaknesses, and strategies to level up.

- Keep that self-reflection train rolling! Analyzing strengths and weaknesses is not a one-time deal, or at least it shouldn't be - it's an ongoing process. Prompt your teenager to make it a habit, like brushing their teeth or checking their Instagram feed. One suggestion is getting together as a family to talk about the good, the bad, and the ugly of the day. This is a great way to stimulate conversation, and talk about ways to work on areas of need, which, done well, can bring out a lot of humorous stories along the way.

- Embrace the quirks and talents that make you unique. Each teenager has a special blend of qualities and skills that make them stand out. Help them see the beauty in their individuality and celebrate their unique strengths. Remind them that these are what set them apart and give them the power to embrace them.

- Weaknesses? More like growth opportunities! Let's flip the script and turn weaknesses into badges of honor, by advocating to our teenagers the value of embracing their limitations and seeing them as springboards for growth. How? Well, you can help them create action plans and seek support to conquer those challenges and emerge more robust than ever.

- Don't get too comfortable. Strengths and weaknesses change and evolve as teenagers progress in their life. What's a strength today might need a little TLC tomorrow, and a weakness can transform into a strength with some dedication and elbow grease.

Remind them to stay flexible and keep re-evaluating their abilities as they continue on their life path.

Unveiling Hidden Gems: Final Thoughts On Strengths And Weaknesses

What did we learn in this chapter? Well, something, I hope! To quote the late, great, and sorely missed comic Bill Hicks, "What's the point? There has to be a point to all this, right?"

Well, in wrapping up this chapter, let's reflect on a few key takeaways. Firstly, your teenager should be encouraged to partake in self-reflection and assessment, as a regular part of their life development, to help ensure they can adapt and grow by consistently evaluating their abilities, values, and areas for improvement. Self-awareness is a skill!

Secondly, teens, like all people in the world, are individuals with their own wild mix of qualities, talents and tastes, that fluctuate as they progress throughout life. If they didn't? Well, it'd be a pretty boring ride for us all. As such, our teens need to be empowered to embrace their individuality and this zenith can be pursued, reached, and obtained by understanding, developing and furthermore celebrating their unique strengths, and even their weaknesses.

You see, rather than something to avoid, uncovering our weaknesses should be viewed as the start of flexing our muscles for inner growth, and not as waving the white flag of defeat. Our kids should be reminded that assessing weaknesses leads us to our own personal projects that are waiting to be upgraded, kinda like learning any skill, or even leveling up in a video game, it takes time, patience, and practice.

Lastly, remind your teen that strengths and weaknesses are not fixed but evolve over time. Just because you find something to be true at one point in time, does not mean that fact is permanent. It is not the end, but the beginning of a lifelong quest for self-awareness and growth.

Chapter 4: No ifs, buts, or Maybes: Effective Decision Making

Greetings, and welcome to Chapter 4. Allow me to expound on the significance of cultivating your teenager's decision-making abilities. It's only natural to want the best for your child and ensure that they make the right choices in life. However, it's fundamental to understand that in order for them to make wise decisions, they need to learn and practice the art of decision-making on their own.

You see, decision-making is a life skill that helps young people develop autonomy, self-confidence, and responsibility. It's a skill that they will need to navigate the complexities of adult life successfully. Our role is not to make decisions for our teenagers but rather to guide them toward making informed decisions that align with their values and goals. Unless their life goals are theft and armed robbery, of course, in that case, you've already made quite a clusterbump of this whole parenting thing. Anyway, I digress...

Encouraging your teenager to make their own decisions may initially feel uncomfortable, but it's an important part of their growth and development. It allows them to learn from their mistakes and experience the consequences of their actions (don't "protect" them from this). Of course, we can provide guidance, support, and advice, but ultimately, as much of the decision-making process as is safe and responsible should be left up to them.

By giving your teen the space to make decisions, you're empowering them to take ownership of their lives. You're helping them develop critical thinking skills, weigh the pros and cons of different options, and make choices that align with their values. This is a crucial element in building resilience and developing a sense of agency.

Your teenager is growing up, and soon they'll be making important decisions without you. Scary, right? Luckily, when they have the chance to make choices and learn from their mistakes, they become more independent and self-sufficient. And there's no denying it, you can't make all their decisions for them forever, no matter how much you might want to.

But here's the bonus: developing strong decision-making skills also helps them become better leaders. Confidence and self-esteem are vital traits for successful leadership, and these can be built through practicing decision-making skills. When teenagers feel confident in their ability to effectively weigh out pros and cons to ultimately make sound decisions, they're more likely to step up and take on leadership roles.

Therefore, as parents, we must provide opportunities for our teenagers to practice decision making skills and allow them to make mistakes without judgment. By doing so, we can help them become decisive successful leaders in their own right.

The Art Of Decisive Leadership And Why It Matters

The act of making decisions requires a blend of analytical thinking, strategic foresight, and emotional intelligence, and is a crucial aspect of effective leadership.

The art of decisiveness refers to the ability to make firm and timely decisions, even in the face of uncertainty or complexity.

Effective problem-solving is at the heart of decision-making (and Entrepreneurship for that matter). Leaders face numerous challenges and must make timely, well-informed decisions to find effective solutions and overcome obstacles. It's like being a problem-solving ninja, slicing through challenges with precision and agility. (Ah ha! I like that, feels like an even more on-point ninja reference!)

Decisive leaders keep things moving forward and by avoiding indecision and analysis paralysis, decisive leaders create a sense of momentum and drive.

Innovation thrives on decision-making. Leaders who embrace it as a catalyst for change and growth inspire their teams to think outside the box and explore new possibilities.

Accountability and responsibility are also demonstrated through decision-making, and leaders who stand by their decisions show integrity and take ownership of outcomes.

That breads trust and credibility and by gaining trust, others believe in your judgment and guidance.

In the competitive landscape of business, opportunities arise and fade quickly. Decisive leaders possess the agility to recognize and seize these opportunities. They understand the value of being proactive and taking calculated risks, enabling their organizations to stay ahead of the curve.

Alright, you ready for some real talk, folks? In the cutthroat world of business, the game is all about snatchin' up those fleeting chances before they're gone in a puff of smoke. Only the sharpest leaders possess the agility to recognize and seize these opportunities. They make miracles happen by taking chances and shaking things up. They understand the value of being proactive and taking calculated risks and keeping that damn curve in their rear view mirror.

Honing decision-making skills involves continuously seeking opportunities for growth and learning. Leaders can engage in activities such as seeking diverse perspectives, soliciting feedback, and actively reflecting on past decisions. In leadership, humility reigns supreme. A truly effective leader understands that they don't hold unrivaled wisdom on every subject that comes their way, be it through their desk or inbox. Seeking the input of a trusted circle of advisors, whom I fondly call "minions" (just kidding) is a valuable practice to ensure clarity when faced with a pressing matter.

These practices enhance their ability to make sound judgments, evaluate alternatives, and navigate complex situations effectively. This has a knock on effect of empowering team members to embrace their own decision-making capabilities and contribute their unique insights and expertise to the collective success of the organization.

Decoding The Decision-Making Journey: Nurturing Teenagers To Become Confident Decision Makers

When it comes to raising teenagers, it's paramount to recognize the value of effective decision-making skills. Teenagers can develop a sense of self-sufficiency and independence that will serve them well throughout their lives when they learn this skill, and by providing opportunities to practice decision-making in tricky situations, parents can help teenagers develop this skill.

Teenagers are wired to seek out social connection: In a podcast interview with Rich Roll, Dr. Andrew Huberman explained that teenagers are in a phase of development where their brains are highly attuned to social connection and approval from peers. This is in part, due to the fact that during adolescence, the brain undergoes significant changes in the regions that govern social cognition and decision-making. As a result, teenagers may be more likely to engage in risky behavior in order to gain social status or approval.

Research supports the idea that encouraging decision-making in teens is vital for their development, a study published in the National Library of Medicine found that teens who had more decision-making autonomy were less likely to engage in risky behaviors, as processes that inform decision-making are uniquely amplified during adolescence, such as, learning from direct experience, reward reactivity, tolerance of ambiguity, and context-dependent orientation toward risk in exciting or peer-laden situations (aka. With their friends).

Moreover, encouraging decision-making in teenagers enables them to develop a greater sense of responsibility and accountability. When they are given the opportunity to make choices and experience the consequences of those choices, they learn to take ownership of their decisions and become more confident in their ability to handle the challenges that life throws their way. This can help them become more resilient and adaptable individuals who are better equipped to handle stress and uncertainty.

Here are some reasons why it's imperative to instill decision-making in teens:

- Builds confidence: Letting teenagers make their own decisions can work wonders for their self-esteem and confidence. Allowing them to flex their decision-making muscles helps them build independence and develop their identities as separate individuals from their parents. When they're given the chance to call the shots, they get a sense of control over their lives and a boost in self-confidence. Plus, if they make good choices, it reinforces their belief in their abilities and helps them easily tackle future challenges. And even if they make a wrong move, they can learn from their mistakes and grow from the experience.

Allowing teens to make decisions can teach them resilience and how to get back up when life knocks them down, which is a critical skill for success.

- Develops critical thinking: Let's face it, we all make bad decisions. But when we embolden teenagers to make their own choices, we're actually helping them develop critical thinking skills. They learn to weigh their options and consider the consequences of their actions, which is a valuable skill not just for avoiding bad haircuts or questionable fashion choices, but also for navigating life's trickier situations. By learning to think critically, teenagers can become savvy problem-solvers and decision-makers, making informed choices and seeing things from different perspectives.

- Promotes independence: As our young teens start to spread their wings and fly the coop, it's time for them to take on more responsibility and learn how to adult. I haven't written Adulting 101, yet, but promoting independence is like a crash course of said book. Making important choices, they'll learn to take ownership of their actions and start thinking about the consequences of their decisions, it's a rite of passage into the real world, where they learn to navigate life's challenges and become responsible members of society.

- Reduces risk-taking behavior: Well, well, well, look at that - research has shown that when teenagers have more say in making decisions, they're less likely to get into all sorts of shenanigans like drug use, alcohol abuse, and risky sexual behavior. That's why it's so pivotal for parents to spur their teens on to make decisions, so they can develop the skills and confidence they need to make responsible choices and avoid all that wacky stuff. And trust me, as someone who's made some questionable decisions in my life, it's much better to make informed choices than to learn the hard way.

So, let's dive into some practical steps that can help us foster a decision-making mindset in teens and guide them on the path to becoming confident and capable leaders. Here are a few strategies that have worked for me and my family:

1.   Offer choices: the power to rule the kingdom of their decisions!

Many of us, as teenagers, didn't have much control over our lives. Our parents made most of the decisions for us, like what to wear, what to eat, and even what time to go to bed. But now, as parents, we have the power to change that for our own teens. By giving them choices, we're not only teaching them how to make decisions, but we're also giving them a sense of control over their own lives. Who knows, maybe they'll even start choosing healthier food options and stop wearing those questionable outfits.

Becoming decisive is a muscle that must be worked. Whenever possible, give your teenager the opportunity to make choices and decisions. This could be as simple as letting them choose the restaurant for dinner or giving them a say in which movie to watch. Or, for instance, you can let them choose what activities they want to do on the weekends or what extracurricular activities they want to pursue. By giving them these choices, you're providing them with the opportunity to consider the options available to them, weigh their pros and cons, and come to their own conclusions, and thus flexing that muscle.

In my own experience, I found that giving my son Noah the freedom to choose his own outfits for school helped him develop his early decision-making skills. Although, at first, he made some wacky fashion choices, he gradually learned what worked well together and started making more thoughtful choices. Now, he even helps me choose my own outfits!

2.   Inspire problem-solving: like a detective on a mission to solve the case!

When your teen faces a problem or challenge, instead of immediately providing a solution, ask them to brainstorm solutions and weigh the pros and cons of each option. This will help them learn how to analyze situations, think critically, and make decisions based on their own judgment.

One time, Noah was having trouble with a school project. Instead of giving him the answers, I asked him questions that helped him identify the problem and develop his own solutions. By the end of our conversation, he had a plan that he was excited to execute on his own.

Problem-solving involves identifying an issue or challenge, brainstorming possible solutions, and evaluating and selecting the best course of action.

Here are some practical ways to encourage problem-solving in teenagers:

- Identify the specific problem: When it comes to fruitful problem-solving, one essential step is to identify the specific problem and focus on it. By honing in on the core issue at hand, teenagers can direct their efforts, and by maintaining focus on the particular problem, it will help them develop more efficient and successful resolutions.

- Ask open-ended questions: When your teenager encounters a problem, ask open-ended questions to help them consider different options. This could be as simple as asking, "What are some possible solutions to this problem?" or "What do you think would happen if you chose this option?"

- Promote creativity: Creativity plays a vital role in problem-solving by enabling individuals to explore alternative possibilities and envision new pathways. It inspires teenagers to think beyond the obvious and challenge conventional thinking. By fostering a creative mindset, teenagers can tap into their imaginations, break free from preconceived notions, and generate unique solutions to complex problems.

- Provide guidance: While fostering independence and autonomy in problem-solving is valuable, providing guidance and support to teenagers is equally constructive. As parents or mentors, you can play a fundamental role in helping them navigate the complexities of decision-making and problem-solving by offering perspective, considering pros and cons, and providing advice when needed.

Research has shown that problem-solving skills are critical for success in school, work, and life in general. A study published in the Journal of Educational Psychology found that students who were taught problem-solving skills were more successful in their academic work and were better able to handle stress. Another study published in the Journal of Youth and Adolescence found that problem-solving skills were positively related to academic achievement and social competence.

To put it simply, developing problem-solving skills in teenagers is a vital aspect of their growth and future accomplishments. We can foster this skill by posing questions that elicit creative solutions, exhibiting problem-solving ourselves, fostering creativity, and offering guidance. Studies reveal that having effectual problem-solving abilities leads to academic and social aptitude and triumph in life overall.

3.   Teach decision-making skills: teach them the Jedi ways of making decisions

Here's a fun way to teach your teenager about decision-making skills: Just talk to them! Share your own decision-making process and show them how you consider all the angles before making a choice. Not only will they appreciate the wisdom you're dropping, but they'll also learn how to think critically and make informed choices. And let's face it, it's not every day that teenagers listen to their parents, so you might as well take advantage of this opportunity to teach them something valuable! I like to involve Noah in choosing which home improvement projects to tackle next or where to go on vacation. I explain my thought process as we discuss different options and always give him a say in the final decision. It's been great to see him learn from these experiences and develop his own capacity for critical analysis often providing excellent view points I never considered.

Research has shown that involving children in decision-making can have a positive impact on their development in a multitude of ways. A study published in the Journal of Family Psychology found that children who were involved in family decision-making had higher self-esteem, better problem-solving skills, and a greater sense of responsibility.

4.   Let them fail forward: Let them make mistakes

Ah, yes, the inevitability of mistakes. It's like that old saying quoted by Tyler Durden in Fight Club, "you can't make an omelet without cracking a few eggs." Similarly, you can't learn how to make good decisions without making some bad ones. it can be tempting to shield our teenagers from making mistakes, but that's not doing them any favors. In fact, it's important to let them make their own decisions, even and especially when we think they might be wrong. This allows them to build resilience and learn from their experiences. So, don't be afraid to let them stumble and fall - it's all part of the journey.

I remember Noah wanting to buy a new video game with his allowance money. I thought it was a waste of money, but I let him make the decision on his own. After he bought the game, he realized it wasn't as fun as he thought it would be and regretted his choice. But he learned a practical lesson about the importance of considering his options before making a hasty purchase.

Allowing your teenager to make decisions can be a valuable way to help them learn how to weigh their options and make informed choices. Encouraging problem-solving skills can also help them develop resilience and learn from their mistakes. By teaching them how to make decisions based on what they think is best, you're helping them become more independent and confident in their abilities. Ultimately, the goal is to help them become self-sufficient leaders who are capable of making their own decisions and navigating the challenges of adulthood.

5.   Spread their wings: Foster independence

Encouraging your teenager to take on more responsibility and make decisions independently is a key part of their development. Some practical ways to encourage your teenager to take on more responsibility:

Give them control over their own finances. This could involve giving them an allowance or helping them to open a bank account. Enliven them to budget and save their money and involve them in decisions about how to spend it.

Let them plan their own schedule: Galvanize your teenager to take responsibility for their own time by letting them plan their own schedule. Mistakes along the way, that's just character-building material for their future memoir.

6.   Provide guidance: Don't let them wander in the dark

It's a fine line to walk between allowing our teenagers to make their own decisions and being there to offer guidance and support. Just telling them to make decisions and then leaving them to their own devices is like sending them on a road trip with no GPS or map - it's a disaster waiting to happen.

So, what can you do? Well, you can help them navigate the road of life by providing some guidance along the way. For example, suppose they're considering attending a party where there may be some questionable substances. In that case, you can offer some insight into the potential risks involved. And if they're still unsure, you can remind them that they have a secret weapon: you!

Let them know you're always there to offer advice, support, or a listening ear. They can come to you with any questions or concerns they may have, and you'll be their wingman, ready to help them tackle any obstacles that come their way.

Remember, providing guidance doesn't mean making decisions for them. It's about helping them develop their own analytical skills, and developing their process while you're there supporting them. You're helping them become more independent and self-reliant, while also ensuring that they have the tools they need to make smart choices in life.

So, how can you put this into practice and help your teen? Here are some practical ways to offer guidance and support:

- Help them consider the consequences of their choices: Empower your teenager to consider the potential outcomes of their choices, by discussing with them the potential consequences of different decisions, and help them weigh the pros and cons. Have them visualize running the tape forward in their mind. Ask them, "If you choose that option, what could happen next? And if that happened, what would it lead to after that?" Sometimes seeing the chain of consequences a couple links down the line is a more powerful motivator for avoiding risky behavior or encouraging delayed gratification for a bigger pay out later on.

- Offer advice when needed: If your teenager is struggling to make a decision, offer guidance and support. Maybe help them to make a pros v cons list, or share your own experiences, help them tune into their intuition and gut feeling, as well as offer advice on how you approach the decision-making process.

- Celebrate their successes: When your teenager makes a good decision, celebrate their success, continue to praise their efforts and endorse them to continue making responsible choices. What we put our attention on expands and therefore it's important we direct adequate focus on the elements our younguns do well. Let's catch them being good and validate them when their choices pay off!

- Encourage open communication: Create an environment where your teenager feels comfortable talking to you about their decisions and seeking your advice. Promote open communication, and be willing to listen and offer support when needed.

A Story About Noah

Coming up against yourself is the real game. And every time we do, we love ourselves a little more. Any developmental exercise laid out in this book has a specific purpose (obviously), which is mainly to develop a particular skill or cultivate a specific mindset. However, there is a deeper, arguably more significant, and profound phenomenon at play here; In stretching for that skill, your future leader will come face to face with resistance. This is worthy of inspection.

When needing to give a public speech, that resistance may present itself as a lump in your throat, the true indicator and physical manifestation of the fear caused by the plethora of potential outcomes. Particularly, the possibility your mind seems to love offering, in an unsolicited fashion, that this may not just go terribly, but be the last speech you ever give, all while your body appears to be seamlessly cooperating on a biological level with the terrifying notion. Oddly, apparently, more people are afraid of public speaking than death.

While attempting to practice your active listening exercises and pay attention deeply, resistance may show up as the anxiousness, bouncing knee, and wondering mind screaming to let you out of a conversation that couldn't possibly be any more effective at eliciting the type of deep, suffocating, mental claustrophobia that only true pointlessness can warrant.

Before stepping on the mat for a fight, it's the surging heart rate, cortisol flooding your veins, and heightening your respiratory rate with the express evolutionary purpose of temporarily increasing your strength and speed. A neat little adaptive trick of evolutionary biology designed to stack the survival odds in our favor should our poor naked predecessors find themselves being chased by a bear through the woods. Your body yells "RUN!". Your brain asking why on earth you were crazy enough to sign yourself up for this experience ON PURPOSE!

Sometimes the resistance comes in the form of crippling depression. The psychological burden experienced from a chemical imbalance, or life dealing a few too many consecutive blows in a row (also leading to chemical imbalance). That proverbial weighted blanket feeling like 1,000 pounds pressing down on every inch of you until your poor little cells wanna pop. You need to go work, but just the shower seems impossibly far... miles and miles away, and slipping further.

The objective may seem like crushing the aforementioned speech, developing the communication skills you have been practicing, standing on the podium at the competition and receiving your medal, or even just putting your feet on the floor in the morning and getting out of bed, and in one sense it is. It IS because developing the skills, or even better, putting these developed skills to the test, builds competence and write this one down…

COMPETENCE CREATES CONFIDENCE

However, in another sense, the resistance itself is the key. The resistance brings you an opportunity to face yourself. To overcome yourself. I say "Yourself" because the resistance is not some outside force. The resistance is a part of you. That lump in your throat, the fear that's just trying to protect, the impatience. These unintegrated elements of the self are your opportunity to exercise agency over the way you handle yourself and, thus, your life. The difficulty creates a choice point. Instead of going through life reactive, chasing pleasure, or avoiding pain (both of which I have done plenty of mind you), you get to proactively transcend your biological and evolutionary impulses to a position of sovereignty. To provide yourself the opportunity to ask yourself the following questions:

"How do I feel?" And, "What am I committed to?"

The first question creates mindfulness and awareness. The bigger the resistance or feeling, the more important it is to acknowledge and experience it. We're not trying to build numb productivity robots here. And we certainly don't want these feelings suppressed only to build up until they inadvertently and unexpectedly erupt at some undoubtedly less-than-convenient time in the future.

Presence is powerful. Eckart Tolle wrote many books on the subject, primarily The Power of Now (a staple of my childhood and a must-read in my not-so-humble opinion). Nevertheless, if you want an emotion to build, don't acknowledge it. If you'd like it to dissipate, acknowledge it. Check in with what you're experiencing. Is it emotional or physical? Where in your body is it? When you've properly acknowledged it, ask yourself the second and more powerful question: "What am I committed to?". Then, and only then, do you make your behavioral choice.

To take our earlier example of Noah giving the speech after his fundraiser, he demonstrated this mechanism very young. He'd hold out one hand palm up like he was attempting to scoop water and ask, "How am I feeling?". Looking at his hand, he said, "I'm scared. My heart is beating really fast! My hands are shaky and a little tingly. I'm also excited and happy!"

"Good Noah! Now, what are you committed to?"

Holding out his other hand, now both palms up, and says, "Ummmmm," pausing thoughtfully and adorably, "I want to be really good at speaking."

"Anything else, beautiful boy?" I've always been able to be sincere with him, so I don't mean it patronizingly when I say I was struggling to withhold my smile while choking on my parental joy watching him adorably apply this practice. I think the Yiddish word my grandparents would have used was "kfel", and I should probably look up that spelling.

"I want to give a badass speech, and I wanna have fun!"

"Awesome! So, what are you going to do?" I said in the same tone of voice I would have used to ask myself while self-parenting (a regular practice for me to this day).

"I'm gonna go do that."

"Amazing."

You all know how this turned out, his elementary school aforementioned accolades notwithstanding, this is one of the strongest muscles you can possibly build. In yourself, your teen, or in a leader of any age. The ability to feel and act anyway.

The habit of creating awareness. The habit of instantly re-directing the focus to your goal or objective as soon as the underlying "feeling" surfaces. The ability to be, and live, vision-driven. What could possibly be more imperative to one's capacity to lead than creating clarity of commitment, the courage to follow it, and a clear vision for others to follow?

Final Thoughts On Fostering Decision Making Skills

In a world where teens are constantly bombarded with information and choices, it's imperative to teach them how to navigate through it all. Encouraging decision-making is not just about giving them the freedom to choose, but also about instilling in them the skills and confidence needed to make those decisions. By giving them choices, we are allowing them to practice decision-making, which in turn helps them build their analytical skills and ability to weigh options.

Problem-solving is a critical component of decision-making. By encouraging our teens to brainstorm solutions and analyze situations, we are helping them develop critical thinking skills that they will need for the rest of their lives. And as they develop these skills, we can slowly begin to foster independence in them, allowing them to take on more responsibility and make more complex decisions.

Here's the dichotomy in raising our teenagers, that requires a balanced approach: we want them to spread their wings and make their own decisions, but we also want them to avoid any major catastrophes. We need to master the art of walking the tightrope between giving them freedom to choose and being the ever-present "helpline" when things go haywire. Picture us as their trusty sidekicks, the pros and cons list-makers, diligently guiding them through life's decision-making obstacle course. And hey, even if it means being their personal human Google search engine, we're up for the task! After all, we want their lives to be a series of hilarious misadventures rather than an eternal loop of chaotic confusion.

Research has shown that encouraging decision-making in teens leads to positive outcomes, such as reduced risk-taking behavior and increased self-esteem. As such, we must make a conscious effort to teach our teens this valuable skill. By offering choices, helping them evaluate the possible outcomes and people affected by their choices, encouraging problem-solving, and providing guidance, we can help them become confident and capable decision-makers, ready to take on whatever challenges come their way.

Chapter 5: You Got This - Building Confidence

Now, I know what you're thinking: "Teenagers as leaders? Are you kidding me? They can barely make it through a day without losing their phone or forgetting their homework." Mind you, it is also possible I am projecting as I constantly seem to be misplacing my phone...But either way, hold your horses, if you even have a horse, because here's the deal: In the realm of personal growth and leadership development, confidence is the ingredient that transforms ordinary teenagers into extraordinary leaders.

Think about it. When someone exudes confidence, they have an aura that draws people in. It's like they're wearing a t-shirt that says, "I know what the hell I'm doing, and you should too." And in my experience, that kind of energy is contagious. When teenagers radiate confidence, they inspire trust, motivate others, and become the heroes of their own stories.

"A leader is one who knows the way, goes the way, and shows the way."

- John C. Maxwell

Confidence doesn't just magically appear out of thin air. It's not like a unicorn that poops rainbows and sparkles. No, confidence is something that needs to be nurtured and cultivated, like a delicate plant that grows stronger with each beam of sunlight and drop of water. And that's where we come in as the wise and slightly exhausted adults in the room. It is our responsibility as adults to support and guide our teenagers in their journey toward unlocking their full potential.

We do this by nurturing their confidence, offering words of encouragement, and, yes, even engaging in the occasional cringe-worthy dance move. Together, we embark on this mission, step by step, as we witness our teenagers grow into the confident leaders they were destined to be.

"The question isn't who's going to let me, it's who's going to stop me."

- Ayn Rand

Time for some serious talk about building confidence in your teenager. Let's confront the reality, building confidence in your teenager is not for those who are faint of heart. It's a bit like trying to teach a cat how to dance - it takes a lot of patience, a lot of practice, and a whole lot of tuna. If that doesn't convince you that you're in safe hands (then quite frankly, I don't know what will), fear not. I'm here to guide you through this journey, and to give you the tools, the strategies, and the sharp remarks you need to help your teenager become a walking, talking fireball of confidence. And trust me, when your kid is strutting down the street, head held high, you're going to feel like the proudest parent in the world.

Why Confidence Is Important In Leadership

Let's touch on why confidence is absolutely vital for effective leadership. And no, it's not just because it looks cool when you strut into the office like you own the place (although that is a pretty sweet perk).

When leaders are confident, they inspire their team to be the best versions of themselves, and that leads to some pretty impressive results. It's like a domino effect. Your confidence inspires your team, and their confidence feeds off of yours, and before you know it, you're all crushing it.

And let's not forget, as a leader, you're gonna face some situations that make you want to curl up in the fetal position and cry. But when you're confident, you can make those tough calls. You trust your instincts, and you know you've got this. It's like walking on hot coals (which I've actually done at the aforementioned Tony Robbins seminar "Unleash the Power Within") - you're a little scared, but you know you can handle it.

Last but in no ways least, building confidence in your team members is like planting a garden of success. When you uplift them to take on challenges and support them every step of the way, they start to believe in themselves and grow. And when they believe in themselves, they're more likely to step up and take on more responsibility and maybe even step into leadership roles and achieve even more success. Building confidence in yourself and your team is the key to being a kickass leader.

How To Build Confidence In Your Teen

If you're up for the challenge, let's embark on this exhilarating journey together. We'll equip your teenager with the tools and mindset to embrace their unique greatness, fostering unwavering confidence along the way. Let's get ready to witness our teen's transformation into a remarkable force, radiating self-assurance and blazing their own trail toward success:

1.   Encourage positive self-talk

We've all been there. That negative voice in your head that tells you you're not good enough, not smart enough, not cool enough... you get the idea. And unfortunately, that voice can really mess with your confidence. Teens often have negative self-talk, which can lead to a lack of confidence. So, if you've got a teen in your life, and I presume you do as you've read this far! Here's what you need to do: Motivate them to speak positively about themselves and their abilities. This can be challenging, but it's important. Remind them of their strengths and achievements, and help them reframe those negative thoughts into something positive. It's worth it. Because when you believe in yourself, when you speak kindly to yourself, amazing things can happen.

2.   Encouraging self-discovery and self-acceptance

In the quest to build confidence in our teenagers, we must guide them toward self-discovery and help them uncover their unique strengths, interests, and values.

One such way to build confidence is a delve into the world or motivation, whether it be intrinsic (internal) motivations that we are driven to pursue simply for joy and genuine appreciation, or extrinsic (external), which might include benefits such as money, course credits and so on. In short, our performance is motivated by three essential factors: autonomy, competence, and relatedness. To read more about intrinsic motivation and Self-Determination Theory, I highly recommend checking out the free resources and exercises, which are too numerous to list here, at Positive Psychology (www.positivepsychology.com).

We can embolden them to try new activities, explore different hobbies, and embark on adventures that ignite their curiosity. We cheer them on as they dabble in various pursuits, from painting to coding, from sports to theater. We let them roam freely in the garden of self-discovery, watering the seeds of their potential and watching them blossom.

3.   Provide difficult opportunities for success

Let me give you some advice on how to build up that confidence muscle. It's about giving your teen opportunities to try new things and succeed! Whether it's picking up a new hobby, taking on a new responsibility, or setting a goal and achieving it, each success will help them believe in themselves just a little bit more. So don't be afraid to fortify them to take risks, challenge themselves, and push outside of their comfort zone. Who knows what amazing things they can accomplish? And when they do succeed, take a moment to celebrate! They deserve it. Keep that momentum going, and before you know it, they'll be unstoppable.

4.   Celebrate accomplishments

Whether they got an "A" on a test or became a master of a new skill, giving them props and celebrating their accomplishments is key. Whether it's a small victory or a grand achievement, we need to make sure we shine a spotlight on their successes. This is a surefire way to boost their self-esteem and let them know they're capable of achieving great things.

But it's not just about external validation. We also teach them the art of self-recognition. We help them develop the ability to pat themselves on the back and appreciate their own achievements. We remind them that their efforts and progress deserve their own applause, their own standing ovation.

In this process, we foster a sense of accomplishment and self-belief within them. They start to internalize their successes, building a reservoir of confidence that fuels their future endeavors.

5.   Applaud risk-taking

True growth and confidence lie just beyond the boundaries of familiarity. Aim to instill in your teenager the belief that in those moments of uncertainty and vulnerability, they have the potential to discover their hidden talents, passions, and strengths.

Share your inspirations and favorite stories of great leaders and innovators who encountered failure, yet persevered and emerged stronger and wiser. In doing you'll equip them with an attitude that embraces challenges and setbacks as catalysts for growth and innovation. Maybe you're a huge David Goggins fan? Great, share that and encourage them to read his book, or maybe Warren Buffet inspired you to educate yourself in becoming financially literate, cool, pass that on.

In this process, they learn through you and others, to be resilient, adaptable, and resourceful. They'll begin to understand that it is through failure that they can uncover their true potential, refine their skills, and forge their own unique paths.

6.   Model confident behavior (not know it all behavior)

You are a walking, talking example of how to be confident (or not so confident, if that's the case) for your teenager. So, if you want your teen to have confidence, don't be afraid to take healthy risks and step out of your comfort zone, even if it means embarrassing yourself a little. Be bold to approach new people and start a conversation, take on a challenge at work, or sign up for a physical challenge that shows you're not afraid to stretch yourself, be it a 5k run, a triathlon or whatever.

Your teen is watching, and they'll see it's okay to be imperfect and take chances. And who knows, maybe you'll even surprise yourself and accomplish something great! So go ahead, be a confident role model, and watch your teen follow in your footsteps.

In the annals of rock 'n' roll history, few names shine as brightly as that of Paul McCartney, the iconic musician and former member of The Beatles. While the world knew him as a prolific songwriter and charismatic performer, his greatest accomplishment lay in his extraordinary bond with his daughter, Stella McCartney.

Throughout Stella's formative years, Paul recognized the importance of nurturing her self-belief. He understood that confidence wasn't something one could simply bestow upon another like an extravagant gift; it needed to be cultivated from within. And so, with unwavering dedication, Paul embarked on a mission to help his daughter discover and harness her own inner strength.

One of the ways Paul instilled confidence in Stella was through his unwavering support of her creative endeavors. From an early age, Stella exhibited a keen interest in fashion design. Recognizing her passion and talent, Paul wholeheartedly embraced her chosen path, encouraging her to explore her creativity and pursue her dreams.

In an industry known for its fickle nature and cutthroat competition, Paul stood by Stella's side, providing a steadfast pillar of support. He attended her fashion shows, showcasing his unmistakable smile as he watched her designs come to life on the runway. His presence was a testament to his unwavering belief in her abilities, bolstering her confidence and inspiring her to push boundaries in her craft.

Beyond the public displays of support, Paul engaged in intimate conversations with Stella, fostering a sense of empowerment within her. He listened attentively to her ideas and dreams, offering guidance and wisdom along the way. Through these conversations, Paul imparted his own life lessons and encouraged Stella to trust her instincts and make decisions with conviction.

As Stella embarked on her own fashion label, she faced inevitable challenges and setbacks. Yet, Paul remained her rock, providing her with a much-needed anchor during turbulent times. He shared stories of his own triumphs and failures, reminding her that resilience and self-belief were the cornerstones of success.

One particular instance exemplified Paul's commitment to boosting Stella's confidence. When her designs were met with skepticism by industry insiders, Paul's response was unequivocal. He proudly wore his daughter's creations, effortlessly flaunting them at public events and red-carpet galas. His actions spoke louder than any words could. Through this display of unyielding support, he communicated to Stella and the world that her talent was undeniable, further cementing her belief in herself.

Paul McCartney's unwavering commitment to his daughter's growth serves as a poignant reminder of the transformative power of parental encouragement. With his unwavering belief and unfaltering support, he helped foster Stella's confidence, enabling her to navigate the challenging terrain of the fashion industry with resilience and grace.

Today, Stella McCartney stands tall as a renowned fashion designer in her own right, an embodiment of the confidence and self-assurance instilled in her by her beloved father. Her journey stands as a testament to the profound impact a famous figure can have on their child's self-belief, offering inspiration to parents and children alike.

In the symphony of life, Paul McCartney's unwavering support of Stella McCartney serves as a harmonious reminder that when we lift others up, when we believe in their potential and nurture their confidence, we create a symphony of resilience and achievement that resonates through generations.

Noah's Story

My son Noah struggled with confidence for years. He was always hesitant to try new things and was afraid of failing. I knew I needed to help him build his confidence, but I wasn't sure how.

One day, I decided to roused Noah to try out for the school play. He had always enjoyed acting but had never had the confidence to audition. I reminded him of his past successes in drama class and encouraged him to give it a shot.

To my surprise, Noah auditioned and was cast in a lead role! Watching him perform on stage with confidence and pride was one of our proudest moments up until that point... From that day on, Noah's confidence grew, and he began to take risks and try new things. Today, he is a confident and capable young adult who is ready to take on new challenges with a deeper self-belief.

Final Thoughts On Building Confidence In Our Teens

Confidence is not a destination; it's a journey. As we wrap up our exploration of building confidence in our teenagers, it's important to remember that confidence is not something we achieve and check off our to-do list. It's an ongoing process of self-discovery, self-acceptance, and personal growth.

Building confidence in your teenager is not just a nice-to-have, it's an absolute must if you want them to slay at adulting. You don't want them turning into a nervous wreck at the first sign of a challenge, do you? Nope, you want them to be like the Hulk - confident, fearless, and ready to smash any obstacle in their way.

So, how do you turn your timid teen into a confident powerhouse? You need to provide your teen with opportunities to exercise their capacities, explore what motivates them, and to learn. This is an area that really needs some time and attention to sit with them, or encourage them, to complete some self-reflection exercises and see what they drift toward and what gets them in the flow state. Maybe it's signing them up for a club or sport they're interested in trying or encouraging them to take on a challenging project at school.

And, as the famous saying goes, "Nothing ventured, nothing gained." Support your teen to take on new challenges, try new things, and step outside of their comfort zone. When they do, they'll start to see just how capable they really are.

Chapter 6: Teaching Resilience

Welcome, to Chapter 6! Let's get deep into the core of resilience and its momentous role in shaping teenage leaders. A journey that goes beyond the ordinary.

"You may encounter many defeats, but you must not be defeated. In fact, it may be necessary to encounter the defeats, so you can know who you are, what you can rise from, how you can still come out of it."

~ Maya Angelou

Resilience is the real deal, it sets apart the people and leaders who thrive from the ones who crumble under pressure and it's the key to unlocking untapped potential and achieving remarkable feats.

We're not talking about putting on a tough facade or ignoring hardships, but actually about developing an true inner strength that enables us to navigate life's unpredictable twists and turns, to bounce back from failures and setbacks, armed with invaluable lessons and an unwavering determination to keep pushing forward.

Resilience isn't a magical switch you can flip overnight. It's a skill that must be honed and cultivated and revolves around embracing new challenges, learning from our mistakes, and adapting to change.

"Mental toughness and resilience fade if they aren't used consistently… you are either getting better, or you are getting worse. You're not staying the same."

~ David Goggins

When our teens face a challenge, instead of wallowing in self-pity, they need to ask themselves, "What can I do to fix this?" We need to inspire our teens to be problem-solvers, not problem-dwellers.

Part of resilience is knowing where you are going, your North Star, what you want to achieve and how you're going to get there. But to paraphrase the afore-quoted David Goggins, you need to recognize what you don't like about the journey ahead and visualize how you're going to overcome it. We're going to look at goal setting later in this Chapter as it's a hugely important part of building resilience. Tough battles come our way in life, and our insecurities are exposed by our own minds when we're suffering in pursuit of our goals. The ability to overcome them means knowing what you want, where you're going, and what pain you're willing to suffer to get there.

Let's look at an example. Say a teenager, let's call him Josh, struggles with stress and anxiety related to academic pressures and social challenges at school. He's having difficulty concentrating in class and is starting to feel discouraged about his ability to succeed.

Josh's parents and teachers recognize that he's struggling and suggest that he try engaging in regular physical activity, such as running or joining a local martial school. John decides to try out for the school's cross-country team. Throughout the season, he starts to notice some positive changes in his mood and overall well-being.

He finds that running helps to clear his mind and improve his focus. He learns that when he feels like giving up on a run, that it's mostly in his mind, and if he embraces the feeling and keeps going, he can continue way past the point where his mind asks him to give up. He starts to feel more confident in his ability to tackle the challenges he's facing at school. As he continues to train and compete with the team, he also develops a sense of camaraderie and connection with his teammates, which helps to further boost his resilience and overall well-being.

In this example, encouraging Josh to engage in physical activity helps to promote resilience, regulate his stress hormones, improve his mood, and gives him a sense of social connection and belonging.

This important aspect has been discussed by Dr. Andrew Huberman, a neuroscientist and professor of neurobiology at the Stanford University School of Medicine, who has spoken extensively about the role of physical activity in promoting resilience and well-being. Exercise can help to regulate stress hormones, improve mood, and promote healthy brain function. Encouraging teenagers to engage in regular physical activity, such as team sports, martial arts, or running, can be a great way to biochemically give them a leg-up in almost any aspect of life they have the desire to thrive in.

The Significance Of Resilience In Leadership

Anyone with the desire to become a great leader, must cultivate resilience—that ability to keep going even when life knocks you down. As a leader, you'll face more ups and downs than a rollercoaster ride, so being able to bounce back from setbacks is fundamental. It is the foundation upon which all other lasting achievements will be built.

To stay the course, is all about staying calm under pressure, being flexible and adaptable in the face of change, and keeping a positive attitude during difficult times. When a team sees a leader handling adversity confidently, they'll be more likely to follow their lead and keep pushing forward. So rather than just focusing on skills unique to leadership—it's wise to also work on building resilience muscles to become an unstoppable force. Universally.

Leaders who possess this aforementioned tenacity, as the eye of the storm so-to-speak, are better equipped to handle setbacks and challenges without getting derailed or discouraged to the point of stagnation. They can maintain composure and focus on their goals, even when things get tough. As I've told Noah countless times, while learning to drive around difficult turns, it's imperative you focus on the patch of road you are aiming at, as opposed to looking at the wall you are trying not to crash into. This not only calibrates your mind towards vision driven success, but it can help to inspire and motivate your team to stay the course and persevere through difficult times right along with you.

For example, a leader who has faced significant setbacks in their business can use their resilience to develop new strategies and pivot their approach. They can stay focused on the bigger picture, maintain a positive outlook, and inspire their team to stay motivated and engaged. This can ultimately lead to a stronger, more resilient team, not just individuals, better equipped to face future challenges.

Furthermore, problem-solving becomes second nature to resilient leaders. They seem to possess an unwavering belief that there's always a solution, even in the most challenging circumstances (and despite what their natural human emotions may be indicating). They don't shy away from complex problems. Instead, they thrive in finding innovative and creative ways to overcome obstacles. Their resilience fuels their perseverance, enabling them to navigate the most intricate puzzles and emerge victorious.

Resilience is a vital skill for any leader to have. Here are some examples of how resilience can be important in leadership:

Overcoming failure: As a leader, encountering failure is almost inevitable. But what sets successful leaders apart is their ability to overcome these obstacles and keep moving forward. After all, the difference between winners and losers, that a winner is simply somebody who lost and kept on trying until he or she didn't. This is where resilience comes into play. Resilience enables leaders to face failure head-on and quickly regroup. Rather than becoming bogged down by the disappointment and frustration of a setback (and losing their s**t), resilient leaders use the experience as a learning opportunity. They reflect on what went wrong, identify areas for improvement, and find new strategies for success.

In the pursuit of their goals, leaders encounter failures that can knock them off balance. It's in these moments that resilience reveals its true worth. Without resilience, a leader risks falling prey to discouragement and self-doubt, and ultimately abandoning their aspirations. However, armed with the tenacity that accompanies resilience, a leader maintains unwavering motivation and laser-like focus, allowing them to navigate through even the most formidable obstacles on their journey.

For instance, imagine a CEO launches a new product that fails to gain traction in the market. Rather than giving up, a resilient leader would view this failure as an opportunity to learn (obviously still feeling all the brutal human emotions that naturally arise when something you care about doesn't come to fruition in the expected and desired manner). They might analyze why the product didn't succeed, seek customer feedback, employ a consultant with expertise in an area they've identified as a weak spot, or explore new ways to refine and improve the offering. This could ultimately lead to a better product and a stronger company in the long run.

In short, resilience is imperative for leaders who want to overcome failure and achieve success. By learning from setbacks and staying focused on their goals, resilient leaders can inspire their teams, build a stronger organization, and ultimately achieve greater success. Here are a couple more pertinent points on resilience and leadership:

Handling stress: As a leader, stress is like that annoying person who always shows up uninvited at a party. But like that person, you can't avoid stress in your leadership role (unfortunately, on both counts). The key is to handle it like a pro and maintain your cool even when things get hectic. Resilience is the superhero skill that enables leaders to navigate uncertainty, handle stress, and stay positive despite the chaos around them.

Why is resilience important for leaders when it comes to handling stress? Well, for starters, resilient leaders are better equipped to make sound decisions and inspire their team, even in high-pressure situations that likely have their blood pressure skyrocketing. They know that stress is part of the job, but they don't let it consume them. Instead, they take care of themselves by taking regular breaks, practicing self-care, and seeking support from others when needed.

A resilient leader might even delegate tasks to team members to lighten their workload and prevent burnout. They understand that a healthy leader is a happy leader, and a happy leader is one who can lead their team to success.

In contrast, a leader who lacks resilience might become overwhelmed by stress and make poor decisions as a result. They might lash out at their team, become indecisive, or lose sight of their goals.

By building resilience, leaders can handle stress more effectively, stay focused on their goals, and inspire their teams to do the same. They can create a culture of resilience within their organization, where employees are encouraged to prioritize self-care and support each other during difficult times. Ultimately, this can lead to a more productive, engaged, and resilient team.

Inspiring others: Leadership is not just about achieving individual success but also inspiring and guiding others toward achieving their goals. Resilient leaders—those who have learned to bounce back from setbacks and overcome challenges—are particularly effective at inspiring those around them.

When your team, whether it be your family or community, sees that you can persevere through adversity, they will be more motivated to do the same. This is because resilient leaders demonstrate that challenges and setbacks are not the end of the road but, rather, necessary and unavoidable elements for growth and learning. By modeling resilience, you are building your own success and the success of those around you.

As a parent, you can inspire your teenagers to be resilient by demonstrating resilience in your own life. Talk to your teens about the challenges you have faced, how you overcame them, and what you learned from the experience. What challenges are you facing now? Are you approaching them with a spirit that embodies terminator-esk resilience? If not, pretend your future leader's fate hangs in the balance and your capacity to step up will help them see that setbacks and challenges are a normal part of life and that it is possible to overcome them.

You can also share stories of other resilient individuals with your teens, which opens a gateway to profound discussions about the qualities that define them: unwavering perseverance, contagious optimism, and an expansive growth mentality. These tales become a catalyst for encouraging your teenager to foster these very traits within themselves. By igniting resilience in their hearts, you equip them with an invaluable tool that will shape their lives in remarkable ways.

As they cultivate resilience, your teenagers will not only conquer the challenges and setbacks that life throws their way, but they will also emerge as beacons of inspiration for others. Armed with the strength to rise above adversity, they become a guiding light, empowering and leading those around them toward triumph.

Steps To Cultivate Resilience In Your Teen

Let's get down to business and explore some practical steps. Teaching resilience to our beloved teenagers, is often a tricky task. Still, you can help them develop this important skill with the right strategies.

"Our plans miscarry because they have no aim. When a man does not know what harbor he is making for, no wind is the right wind." ~ Seneca

Thank you, Mr. Seneca, not only for providing sage wisdom and guidance that has remained relevant throughout the ages but also providing the segue into my next point; goal setting.

Help your teenager set realistic goals: Back your teenager to set realistic goals and work towards achieving them, by offering support and guidance as they work towards their goals and help them develop a plan for achieving them. You may have heard of the mnemonic acronym SMART in goal setting. SMART goals are a great framework for anyone to learn and are one of the ways I help Noah set goals.

There is an art to goal setting and the SMART framework which digs into the who, what, why, where and when of goals, as well as, how, is one of the most widely used ways of creating and achieving goals, for very good reason.

To make sure goals are clear and reachable, each one should be:

- Specific (simple, sensible, significant).
- Measurable (meaningful, motivating).
- Achievable (agreed, attainable).
- Relevant (reasonable, realistic and resourced, results-based).
- Time bound (time-based, time limited, time/cost limited, timely, time-sensitive).

I recommend searching online for a resource and some templates with your kid to get the wheels in motion, because setting goals is integral to developing resilience. When your teen has clear goals to work towards, they are better able to stay focused and motivated, even when faced with obstacles. Support your teen to set short-term and long-term goals, while helping them create a plan to achieve them. This can also include:

Setting realistic goals: Assist them in identifying challenging yet attainable objectives that align with their capabilities, desires, and circumstances. By breaking down larger goals into smaller, manageable tasks, they can track their progress and experience a sense of accomplishment along the way. If you can't measure it, you can't manage it. This approach helps them stay motivated and prevents them from feeling overwhelmed or discouraged by setting expectations that are beyond their reach, or results that are beyond their ability to quantify. By fostering the habit of setting realistic goals, you empower your teenager to maintain a positive mindset, persevere through obstacles, and develop the resilience needed to overcome challenges on their path to success.

Break goals down into manageable steps: By chunking larger objectives into manageable tasks, we're turning Mount Everest into a stroll through the park. My Grandfather used to say; "Inch by inch, life's a sinch. Yard by yard, it gets pretty hard". It's all about staying in the moment, embracing the process, and banishing that pesky overwhelm. We want our teenagers to savor every step and bask in the glory of progress. By championing the art of splitting goals into manageable bites, you're handing them a shiny sword of structured thinking. Armed with this mighty weapon, they can face challenges head-on and strut along the path to success like they own the place. Rally the troops and prepare for mini-missions galore, armed with focused determination, and bolstered by accomplishment, your teenager can conquer the world, one manageable step at a time.

Create a plan of action: Collaborate with them to outline a clear roadmap that outlines the necessary steps for reaching their objectives, by setting realistic deadlines for each milestone, which will allow them to stay focused and accountable (primarily, to themselves). Additionally, help them identify the resources and support systems available, such as mentors, teachers, or relevant materials, that can aid them in their progress. Together, they brainstorm strategies and potential challenges they may encounter, equipping them with problem-solving skills and contingency plans. By creating a timeline for accomplishing each step, your teenager gains a sense of structure and direction, fostering a proactive approach to goal attainment independent of mood or motivation level. This planning process instills organizational skills and cultivates resilience as they learn to navigate obstacles, and adapt their strategies as needed. By empowering them to create a solid plan of action, you provide them with the tools and behaviorism necessary to approach their goals with confidence, determination, structure, and skill.

Alright, so now that we've established the destination we're aiming for, it's time to devise some strategies to support our teenagers when they inevitably veer off track. Below are a few additional key insights that can assist in cultivating resilience within your teen:

Foster a growth mindset: When teenagers believe their abilities and intelligence can be developed through hard work and dedication, they are more likely to persevere in the face of challenges and setbacks. (Remember Chapter 3 where we discussed analyzing strengths and weakness and how they are not immovable objects, per se, but can be developed with perseverance and determination).

By contrast, a fixed mindset, which is the belief that one's abilities and intelligence are innate and cannot be changed, can lead to feelings of helplessness and discouragement when faced with difficult tasks or failures. To help your teen develop a growth mindset, it's essential to both model and promote a "growth-oriented" approach to learning and problem-solving. This can also involve:

- Sharing stories: It's time to loosen those emotional screws and embrace vulnerability with a touch of humor. Share a couple of your wild struggles and how you wrestled them down with a combination of blood, sweat, and persistence. This not only models vulnerability and emotional openness but also sends a loud message to your teenager that it's absolutely okay to ask for some backup and support when the going gets tough.

- Praising effort over innate ability: Instead of praising your teen for being "smart" or "talented," focus on praising their effort, persistence, and dedication. This helps to reinforce the idea that hard work and dedication are the keys to success rather than innate ability. Emphasizing the power of "yet". When your teen encounters a difficult task or challenge, incite them to add the word "yet" to the end of their statement. For example, "I can't do this math problem...yet." Or, to use an example a little closer to home; "Stop calling me champ, I haven't won the World Championships... YET!". This helps to shift the focus from their current limitations to their potential for growth and development. Again, focusing on the road they are aiming at, instead of the wall they are trying to avoid. Vision Driven baby!

- Model resilience yourself: When they witness you weathering the storm and bouncing back from setbacks, they're bound to catch those resilient vibes. So, share your battle stories of triumph over adversity and let them see first-hand how you handle life's curveballs. This works particularly well if you share the PRESENT hardships you are dealing with. Here's the thing: your actions as a resilient parent speak volumes. It's like having a megaphone of trust-building and life-skill-equipping powers. By embodying resilience and showing your teen how to navigate the choppy seas, especially while during the voyage, you empower them to do the same both presently and in the future. As ever, it's all about leading by example, my friend.

- Demonstrate problem-solving skills: When confronted with a challenge or setback, it is vital to actively demonstrate problem-solving skills to your teenager. By showcasing your ability to break the problem down into smaller, more manageable parts and developing a well-thought-out plan of action, you effectively model the importance of resilience, perseverance, and determination in overcoming obstacles. Take the time to explain your problem-solving process, highlighting the critical thinking and decision-making involved. This not only teaches your teenager practical problem-solving techniques but also instills the belief that challenges can be tackled with a strategic and positive approach. By openly displaying your resilience and determination, you inspire them to adopt the same mentality when faced with their own difficulties.

- Embrace failure as a learning opportunity: By openly acknowledging and discussing your own failures, you show them that failure is a natural part of the learning process and not something to be feared or avoided. Share stories of your own failures and setbacks, emphasizing how you learned valuable lessons and grew stronger as a result. Encourage your teenager to reflect on their own failures and guide them in finding the lessons within those experiences. By normalizing failure and reframing it as a stepping stone towards growth and improvement, you help your teen develop resilience, adaptability, and an ethos of growth. This approach fosters a healthy attitude towards setbacks. And it empowers them to embrace challenges with a positive outlook, knowing that failure is not the end but an opportunity for personal development and future success.

- Stay positive and optimistic: Cliché as it may appear, there's a reason this one has been pounded into our minds to no end. Let your teenager witness the power of a positive psyche as you tackle each challenge with an unwavering belief that a solution awaits. Rainy day flat tire? Well, at least it's an opportunity for an impromptu dance party while waiting for roadside assistance! As you embody optimism, you cultivate a garden of hope and resilience in your teenager's heart. They see first-hand that setbacks are mere detours on the winding road to success. With the right mindset and attitude, even the mightiest challenges become conquerable mountains. Maybe even containing a hidden pocket of unexpected fun.

Now that we've successfully set a course to nurture a resilient mindset, let's explore how to tend the garden of resilience. As always, I've got you covered with some essential elements and crucial steps on this journey to raising a resilient teenager:

Cultivate a supportive environment: Resilience is not developed in isolation; your teen needs to surround themselves with a network of individuals who offer positive support and guidance. By fostering a supportive environment, you create a safety net for your teenager, helping them stay motivated and on track as they navigate the ups and downs of life. Resilience is not a solo endeavor, but a team effort that thrives within a network of uplifting relationships. What are some ways to achieve this? Let's take a look:

- Encourage positive relationships: Encourage your teenager to build positive relationships with peers, family members, teachers, coaches, and mentors who will provide them with the support and guidance they need. Help them identify and build relationships with people who share their values, inspire them, and can serve as role models. Positive relationships serve as a valuable source of strength and comfort during challenging times, providing a sense of belonging, and a space for them to express their emotions without judgment. Advocate to your teenager the importance of seeking out friends who uplift and inspire them, family members who provide a loving and nurturing environment, teachers who offer guidance and encouragement, coaches who instill discipline and motivation, and mentors who can share wisdom from their own experiences while having qualities your future leader aspires to possess themselves. These relationships contribute to their overall well-being, help them develop a sense of empathy and understanding, and provide a network of support when facing obstacles. By encouraging positive connections, you empower your teenager to build a strong support system to bolster their resilience and provide a solid foundation as they navigate life's journey.

- Be available and present: This one cannot be overstated. Make a conscious effort to be available and present whenever your teen needs someone to talk to, seek advice from, or simply lend a listening ear. Show genuine interest in their life, hobbies, and passions by actively engaging in meaningful conversations. That means meaningful to the both of you. Demonstrate your attentiveness by actively listening and providing supportive feedback (if this is not readily accessible to you, reread the chapter on effective communication). Let them know that their thoughts and opinions are valued and respected. Being responsive to their needs shows that you are there to offer guidance, emotional support, and assistance in finding solutions to their challenges. Your consistent presence and availability create a sense of security and trust, reinforccing to your teen that they have a reliable and caring figure in their life.

- Create a safe space: Establish an environment where they feel comfortable, secure, and free to express themselves. This starts by setting clear boundaries and expectations that promote a sense of structure and stability. Consistency in enforcing these boundaries helps your teenager feel safe and understand what is expected of them. Foster a calm and supportive atmosphere by promoting open communication, actively listening to their concerns, and validating their emotions. Show unconditional love and acceptance by celebrating their individuality and embracing their strengths and weaknesses. Let them know your love is unwavering, regardless of their successes or failures. By creating a safe space, you provide your teenager with a sanctuary where they can develop resilience, knowing they have a loving and supportive home to return to, and a foundation from which they can confidently face life's challenges.

- Celebrate the hell out of their successes: When your teenager achieves something remarkable, it's time to shine the spotlight on their hard work and dedication. As I've said, what you put your attention on expands! Celebrate their triumphs, big and small, with genuine enthusiasm. By acknowledging and honoring their accomplishments, you validate their efforts and send a powerful message: they are capable of achieving greatness. These celebrations boost their confidence, reinforce their belief in perseverance, and inspire them to embrace challenges. Let the festivities begin, and the successes compound!

- Instill healthy habits: Advocate for regular exercise, emphasizing the importance of staying active. Support them to engage in activities they enjoy, whether it's playing a sport, going for a jog, or practicing yoga. In addition to exercise, emphasize the significance of maintaining a balanced diet and making nutritious food choices. At the very least, teach them to read the nutrition facts on the label. Teach them about the benefits of fueling their bodies with whole foods that provide the necessary nutrients for optimal functioning. Moreover, emphasize the importance of getting enough sleep to support their physical and mental health. Help them establish a consistent sleep routine and educate them on the positive effects of quality sleep on their overall well-being...resilience included. By encouraging these healthy habits, you empower your teenager to care for their physical and emotional needs, providing a more stable foundation impervious to outside forces. They will learn that self-care is central to maintaining balance and effectively navigating life's challenges.

- Practice self-care: Show them the importance of prioritizing self-care by incorporating activities that promote your own physical, mental, and emotional well-being. Emphasize the value of restorative sleep, make conscious choices about your diet, and engage in regular physical activities you enjoy, all of which contribute to maintaining overall health and resilience. Additionally, participate in activities that bring you joy and fulfillment, whether it's pursuing a hobby, spending time in nature, practicing mindfulness, or engaging in creative outlets. By prioritizing self-care, you communicate to your teenager that taking care of oneself is not only necessary but also an act of self-respect. It sets a powerful example they can follow in their own lives, encouraging them to develop healthy coping mechanisms for managing stress and challenges.

Now let's get a little esoteric and look beyond the obvious tangibles and at soft skills that have become widely recognized in the world of self-optimization, personal development, stress reduction and staying the course in life and the business world.

Teach coping skills: Resilience also greatly involves knowing how to cope with stress and adversity. Teach your teen healthy coping skills, such as deep breathing, mindfulness, exercise, and journaling. Rally them to find activities that help them relax and recharge.

- Deep breathing: Teaching your teenager to take deep, slow breaths when they feel stressed or overwhelmed is a simple yet effective technique that can significantly benefit their mental and emotional well-being. This practice can help them calm their mind and body, reduce anxiety, and enhance their adaptability when handling stressful situations. When individuals are stressed or overwhelmed, their sympathetic nervous system, responsible for the body's fight-or-flight response, becomes activated. This can lead to increased heart rate, shallow breathing, and a sense of heightened alertness. When activated too frequently, or for too long, it becomes taxing and exhausting on both the mind and body. By intentionally taking deep, slow breaths, your teenager can activate the parasympathetic nervous system, which helps induce a state of relaxation, or at the very least, counterbalances the stress response. When teaching your teenager this technique, it can be helpful to provide them with specific guidance and then practice it together. Galvanize them to find a quiet and comfortable space where they can sit or lie down. Explain the benefits of deep breathing and how it can help them manage stress and anxiety. Guide them to close their eyes, relax their muscles, and take a deep breath in through their nose, counting to four. Then, ask them to hold their breath for a brief moment before exhaling slowly through their mouth, counting to six. Direct them to repeat this cycle several times, focusing on the sensation of the breath entering and leaving their body.By making this a habit, brief as their sessions may be, they will be better equipped to apply deep breathing when facing challenging situations, exams, social pressures, or any other sources of stress. It can improve focus and concentration, enhance self-awareness, and promote a sense of composure.

- Mindfulness: According to the American Psychological Association (AMA), researchers theorize that mindfulness meditation promotes metacognitive awareness, decreases rumination via disengagement from perseverative cognitive activities and enhances attentional capacities through gains in working memory. These cognitive gains, in turn, contribute to effective emotion-regulation strategies.

To introduce your teenager to mindfulness practices, emphasize the numerous benefits they offer, and explain how mindfulness can help them manage stress, reduce anxiety, and enhance their ability to concentrate being fully present in their daily activities. Discuss the scientific research supporting the positive effects of mindfulness on mental and emotional health.

Meditation is a powerful mindfulness practice that involves sitting in a quiet and comfortable position, focusing on the breath, sensations, or a specific object, and observing the thoughts and emotions that arise without getting caught up in them. By teaching your teenager meditation techniques, you provide them with a valuable tool to manage their thoughts and emotions while developing a greater sense of self-awareness. Regular meditation practice can help them become more grounded, centered, and less reactive to stressful situations. Eye of the storm vibes yet again!

Yoga is another form of mindfulness practice that combines physical postures, breathing exercises, and meditation. Encouraging your teenager to participate in yoga classes or follow online tutorials can offer them a holistic approach to mindfulness. Yoga helps to strengthen the mind-body connection and improve flexibility, balance, and posture. It promotes relaxation, reduces muscle tension, and promotes a sense of inner peace and and powerful presence.

Creative outlets: Engaging in creative activities, such as drawing, painting, or playing music, can have a profound impact on your teenager's well-being. These activities offer a range of benefits that extend beyond stress reduction and relaxation, including promoting emotional expression, boosting self-esteem, fostering problem-solving skills, and enhancing cognitive abilities. Creative activities require your teenager to think outside the box, experiment, and find innovative solutions. Uplift your teenager to allocate regular time for creative activities, whether it's by setting up a dedicated art space, providing access to art supplies or musical instruments, or enrolling them in classes or workshops that align with their interests.

Seeking support: Encouraging your teenager to seek support from friends, family members, or a mental health professional when they are struggling to cope with stress or adversity is essential for their overall well-being. It's important to create an environment where they feel comfortable reaching out for help and understand the value of seeking support when needed. If your teenager is experiencing significant distress, it may be beneficial to seek the expertise of a mental health professional. Rouse your teenager to be open to the idea of therapy or counseling as a way to navigate their emotions, develop coping strategies, and gain valuable insights they may not have arrived at on their own. Explain that mental health professionals are trained to provide guidance and support tailored to their specific needs. Help your teenager understand that seeking professional help is a sign of strength and self-care, rather than a sign of weakness. Encouraging them to seek support from friends, family, or mental health professionals demonstrates that their emotional well-being matters, and that they do not have to face challenges alone. By normalizing the idea of seeking help, you empower them to build healthy relationships, develop effective coping strategies, and navigate life's difficulties with the resilience and strength that accompanies community.

Now, I know what you're thinking—these steps sound simple, but implementing them is a journey in itself. And you're absolutely right! But we also have the privilege of empowering our teenagers to embrace challenges, develop effective coping strategies, build supportive networks, and prioritize their well-being. By doing so, we're equipping them with the tools to thrive in an ever-changing world. Feel free to reference this past list as frequently as you feel is necessary.

A Story About Noah

My son Noah has always been a bit of a perfectionist. In elementary school, he put a lot of pressure on himself to get perfect grades, excel in sports, and be popular. One day, he came home from school devastated because he had failed a math test. He was convinced that this one failure would ruin his chances of getting into college (adorable, I know).

I knew this was an opportunity to teach Noah about resilience. I talked to him about the growth mindset and how failure is just a part of the learning process. We worked together to create a plan for improving his math skills, and I encouraged him to keep working hard and not give up. As a parent, it's necessary to model resilience yourself. Show your teen how you handle challenges and setbacks in a positive and productive way. This will help them see that setbacks are a natural part of life and can be overcome with a positive attitude and determination.

Final Thoughts On Teaching Resilience

The importance of resilience in leadership cannot be overstated. Great leaders are often faced with challenging situations and setbacks. A leader who has developed resilience is better equipped to handle these challenges and bounce back from said setbacks. They are able to remain positive and focused, inspire their team, and find creative solutions to problems.

One great example of a leader who demonstrated resilience is Steve Jobs. After being fired from Apple, the company he co-founded, Jobs could have given up. Instead, he went on to start his own successful company, NeXT, which was eventually acquired by Apple in a miraculous chain of events. Jobs returned to Apple and led the company to become one of the most successful technology companies in the world. Through it all, Jobs demonstrated resilience, determination, and an unwavering belief in his vision.

Teaching your teen resilience is an essential aspect of preparing them for leadership. By encouraging them to develop an attitude geared toward growth, teaching them coping skills, encouraging risk-taking, focusing on their strengths, and modeling resilience yourself, you can help them become a confident, leader who is able to navigate challenges and setbacks with poise and precision.

Resilience is not just a temporary fix or a band-aid solution. It certainly is not just about "toughing it out". It's a lifelong journey. As we teach resilience to our teenagers, we must remember that it's not about avoiding challenges, setbacks, or failures. It's about instilling in them the mindset and skills to face these obstacles head-on courageously even shortly after a failure.

"Success is not final, failure is not fatal: it is the courage to continue that counts."

~ Winston Churchill

By embracing challenges and reframing setbacks as opportunities for growth, our teenagers develop an unyielding attitude in the pursuit of success. They learn to adapt, innovate, and persevere, even in the face of adversity. And through this journey, they become not only resilient leaders but also resilient individuals who are equipped to navigate the complexities of life.

Let's take a moment to recap what we just learned about building resilience in our teenage soldiers. Focus on their strengths rather than their weaknesses. Support them to set achievable goals and celebrate their accomplishments regardless of how minuscule they may appear, to fortify your teen to focus on the positives in any situation and help them identify the lessons they can learn from difficult experiences and how they can use these lessons to become better leaders in the future.

Bolster them to take care of their physical, emotional, and mental well-being by engaging in activities such as exercise, meditation, and spending time with friends and family. Inspire your teen to view setbacks as opportunities for growth and to continue working on their resilience skills even when things are going well. When they face a challenge, instead of cowering in fear, they need to ask themselves, "What resources do I have to overcome this challenge?" And when they do overcome a challenge, we need to celebrate, pop some champagne, dance, and make some noise!

Chapter 7: Building Compassionate Teenagers

(aka Promoting Empathy)

Let's explore the importance of empathy and how to promote it in your teen. You may be thinking, "Empathy? Jeez, that sounds like a soft skill that only therapists and hippies care about." And you may be partly correct! But hear me out. Empathy is a critical skill for any leader (and person) to possess.

Think about it, if you're a leader who can't connect with your team members or understand their emotions and experiences, how are you supposed to build trust and inspire loyalty?

When you show empathy, you demonstrate that you value your team members and care about their well-being. And when your team members feel valued and understood, they're more likely to be productive and engaged.

Show your teen that it's okay to talk about their emotions and to be vulnerable, advocate for them to listen actively to others and try to understand their point of view. When your teen practices empathy, they'll not only become a better leader but also a better friend, a better partner, and a better human being.

You play a central role in promoting empathy in your teen. You can start by modeling empathy in your own interactions with others. Show your teen how to actively listen and validate others' feelings, even if you don't necessarily agree with them. Talk these interactions over with your teenager. Try putting yourself in the other person's shoes, and thinking about how they might be feeling and what they might be going through as a discussion exercise. It's easy to jump to conclusions or make assumptions about someone based on their behavior or actions. Try to avoid doing this and instead approach the conversation with an open mind, show others their feelings and points of view are valid and heard. When you lead by example, others will follow suit, including your teen. They will be more likely to treat others with empathy and understanding as well.

If you want your teenager to grow up to be a decent human being, one way you can do that is by encouraging them to volunteer or get involved in community service. I mean, sure, they might grumble and complain about having to spend their Saturdays picking up trash or serving soup to the homeless. Still, it'll be so valuable to them in the long run.

When your kid is elbow-deep in the garbage, they're gonna be exposed to all sorts of people and experiences they might not have had otherwise. They might meet someone who's been dealt a crappy hand in life and realize that not everyone has it as easy as they do. Or they might see first-hand the profound impact a simple act of kindness can have on someone's day.

Plus, it'll give them something to put on their college applications besides their stellar Fortnite stats. So go ahead and champion your teen to volunteer or get involved in community service. Who knows, they might just surprise you and return home with a newfound appreciation for the world around them.

What Makes Empathy Crucial In The Realm Of Leadership?

In the dynamic world of leadership, empathy emerges as a powerful force, transcending boundaries and shaping remarkable outcomes. Empathetic leaders have an uncanny knack for truly grasping the emotions and perceptions of others, enabling them to foster trust, inspire motivation, and cultivate a supportive environment where individuals thrive.

Moreover, empathy plays a crucial role in navigating conflicts, breaking down barriers, and championing inclusivity, ultimately paving the way for meaningful change. When leaders can understand the needs, concerns, and perspectives of their team members, they can make better decisions and take actions that benefit the team as a whole.

Why does empathy hold such significance? Well, it possesses the ability to forge deep connections through enhanced communication, understanding, and collaboration, and thus, helps leaders build trust and establish strong relationships with their team. When team members feel that their leader understands and cares about them, they're more likely to feel motivated, engaged, and committed to the cause or the task at hand. And when conflicts and difficult conversations arise, empathy can help leaders navigate those situations with more grace and understanding to find a beneficial and positive outcome.

But empathy isn't just for leaders. It's for everyone. Teaching your teen to be empathetic can help them become more successful in their personal and professional lives. Empathy is an essential skill for building strong relationships, collaborating effectively with others, and navigating complex social situations.

Now, picture this: you're having a good old-fashioned heart-to-heart with your old man. The kind of wholesome moment that makes you want to sit back, crack open a cold one, and soak up the fatherly wisdom. Maybe it's over a couple of beers or perhaps at a Sunday BBQ. Either way, he's imparting some sage advice in a scene straight out of a feel-good movie, and this is more or less what he says about encouraging empathy:

- Model good communication: To do this, you need to be clear and concise, expressing yourself respectfully, and actively listening to your kid. As Arthur Schopenhauer said, "To use many words to communicate few thoughts, is everywhere the unmistakable sign of mediocrity. To gather much thought into few words stamps the (wo)man of genius."

- Create opportunities for discussion: Help your teenager practice their communication skills by encouraging them to share their thoughts and feelings about different topics. We can ask open-ended questions that promote dialogue and self-expression in a respectful and constructive manner.

- Calm and respectful tone: Maintain a calm and respectful tone when speaking with your teenager, even during disagreements. Avoid raising your voice or using derogatory language. Model respectful language and encourage them to do the same.

- Provide feedback: Praise your teen's efforts and give them specific, constructive feedback on areas for improvement while also encouraging them to keep practicing and developing their skills.

How To Promote Empathy In Your Teen

1. Set a good example: Your teen learns a lot from watching you, so you're literally their empathetic role model, so it's wise to show your teen that you care about others and are willing to listen to their concerns. Try to understand things from their perspective and validate their feelings and show them you care.

2. Nurture perspective-taking: To foster this ability, parents can encourage open and non-judgmental conversations, actively listen to their teenager's experiences and viewpoints, and validate their

emotions and perspectives. Engaging in discussions about different cultures, beliefs, and social issues can broaden their understanding of diverse perspectives. Modeling perspective-taking through our own behavior and being open to hearing and respecting differing opinions can also be influential. Provide opportunities for reflection, challenge stereotypes, and foster an inclusive environment, will help you play a positive role in nurturing their empathic ability and inadvertently promote positive social interactions.

3. Provide opportunities for community service: We can inspire our teens to step into the world of volunteering and community service, where they can embrace a rich tapestry of people and experiences that ignite compassion within them. It's like unlocking a backstage pass to the world, granting them a front-row seat to assorted backgrounds, cultures, and beliefs. Whether they're dedicating their time to community service, volunteering, or participating in cultural exchange programs, we're inviting our teenage leaders to expand their horizons and cultivate empathy. Just imagine them collecting a vibrant collection of empathy badges, each symbolizing a new connection and a profound understanding of the world that surrounds them.

4. Teach active listening skills: We talked about how Noah and I have a saying in our house, "LISTENING IS A SUPERPOWER." We want our

teenagers to be masters of listening, using techniques like paraphrasing, summarizing, and asking open-ended questions. Active listening is a critical component of empathy. It involves fully focusing on the speaker and trying to understand their message. Teach your teen active listening skills, many of which we have covered at length previously, such as making eye contact, nodding, and asking questions to clarify.

5. Discuss emotions and feelings: Embolden your teen to talk about their own emotions and feelings and help them identify and understand the emotions and feelings of others. This can help them develop empathy and emotional intelligence. We want our teenagers to express themselves with the power of empathy, kindness, and respect. By using "I" statements, active affirmation, and validation, they can build bridges of empathy that reach straight to the hearts of others.

6. Practice empathy in everyday situations: Look for opportunities to practice empathy in everyday situations, such as, if you sees someone struggling with a heavy bags at the grocery story, spur your teen to offer assistance and join in yourself, show your teen it pays to be kind and compassionate towards others.

By practicing empathy, teens can establish stronger bonds with their peers, friends, and family. They will also gain the ability to tackle conflicts head-on without any of the awkwardness that accompanies these situations. Moreover, these skills will assist them in becoming more empathetic and compassionate individuals, which is particularly important in today's world. So, if you want to raise your teenager to be a socially adept, empathetic, and communicative person, it's high time you start introducing them to these skills.

Cultivating empathy in your teen transcends effective leadership; it extends to their overall well-being and their ability to live a more fulfilling life. As caring adults nurturing an empathetic nature is a gift that will positively impact every aspect of their lives.

Empathy enables teens to navigate the complexities of human emotions and respond with compassion and sensitivity. When teenagers develop empathy, they unlock a profound understanding of the human experience. They learn to see beyond their own standpoint and connect with others on a deeper level. This ability to empathize fosters meaningful relationships, strengthens social bonds, and enriches their interactions with friends, family, and the wider community.

In addition to enriching personal relationships and fostering self-growth, empathy also expands a teenager's worldview. It opens their eyes to the wide-ranging perspectives, experiences, and challenges faced by people from different backgrounds and cultures. This expanded perspective empowers them to become active global citizens capable of creating positive change and contributing to a more inclusive and equitable society.

A Story About Roald And Lucy Dahl

In the world of literature and imagination, one name shines brightly: Roald Dahl. Renowned for his enchanting stories that captured the hearts of readers, young and old, Dahl's own life embodied the spirit of empathy and compassion. And it was through his own actions that he nurtured these qualities within his own children, leaving an indelible mark on their lives.

One of Dahl's most cherished children was his daughter, Lucy Dahl. As she navigated the ups and downs of her formative years, Roald recognized the importance of empathy in shaping her character. He understood that empathy was not a skill one could merely teach but rather something that had to be experienced and felt on a deeply personal level.

Roald's efforts to instill empathy in Lucy were woven into the very fabric of their everyday lives. As an accomplished storyteller, Roald often regaled his children with tales that transported them to whimsical worlds, where characters grappled with adversity and discovered the power of empathy. Through these stories, he imparted valuable life lessons. And he sparked conversations that nurtured Lucy's understanding of other people's perspectives and feelings.

Beyond storytelling, Roald actively engaged in acts of kindness and compassion, leading by example. He would often involve Lucy and her siblings in various charitable endeavors, encouraging them to volunteer their time and resources to help those less fortunate. Whether it was visiting children in hospitals or supporting local community initiatives, Roald emphasized the importance of extending a helping hand to those in need.

One specific example showcased Roald's commitment to instilling empathy in Lucy. As a young girl, Lucy experienced her fair share of challenges and disappointments. During these trying times, Roald provided her with unwavering support, creating a safe space for her to express her emotions and encouraging her to develop a keen sense of empathy towards herself. By offering understanding and compassion, he laid the groundwork for her to extend that same empathy to others.

Roald also fostered a deep connection with nature, instilling in Lucy an appreciation for the natural world and the creatures that inhabited it. They would spend hours exploring the outdoors, observing the wonders of the natural environment. Roald encouraged Lucy to treat every living being with respect and compassion, fostering a sense of empathy that extended beyond human relationships.

These experiences left an indelible mark on Lucy, shaping her into a compassionate and empathetic individual. As she embarked on her own path in life, she carried with her the invaluable lessons instilled by her father. Lucy went on to establish her own philanthropic initiatives, dedicating herself to causes that championed empathy, kindness, and social justice.

Roald Dahl's commitment to fostering empathy within his daughter stands as a testament to the transformative power of compassion. Through his stories, acts of kindness, and unwavering support, he instilled in Lucy a deep understanding of others' emotions and experiences. Roald's legacy lives on through Lucy's endeavors as she continues to inspire others to cultivate empathy and make a positive impact on the world.

In the tapestry of life, Roald Dahl's efforts to nurture empathy in his child serve as a poignant reminder that our ability to understand, empathize, and connect with others lies at the heart of our shared humanity. And as we embrace empathy, we create a ripple effect of compassion that has the power to shape a more empathetic and understanding world.

Final Thoughts: The Power Of Empathy In Leadership

Empathy takes center stage in the symphony of leadership, playing a powerful melody that resonates with understanding, compassion, and connection. As we conclude our exploration of promoting empathy in our kids, let's take a moment to appreciate the profound impact it has on their growth and the world around them.

By cultivating empathy, teens become attuned to the needs, desires, and struggles of those around them. They become better equipped to serve and add value to whoever or whatever they come in contact with, and the world will reward them accordingly. Especially as they develop a keen sense of understanding that transcends superficial judgments and empowers them to make decisions that consider the collective welfare. Through empathy, leaders create an environment where everyone feels seen, heard, and valued, fostering a culture of inclusivity and respect – and that's what we're seeking to foster in our kids.

Let's get our kids curious about active listening, empathy-building exercises, and igniting a genuine hunger to understand others' perspectives, so our teens can go deep down the rabbit hole of human connection which simultaneously comes with a treasure trove of understanding. When our teenagers grasp this, they can begin inspiring others through their actions, proving that kindness and understanding are not weaknesses but kickass strengths that take their life, and leadership game, to a whole new level. They'll be the cool kids on the empathy block, leading the way with hearts full of compassion and minds open to the beautiful tapestry of human experiences.

Chapter 8: Cultivating a Positive Mindset

Life can be tricky sometimes (understatement of the century), and welcome to Chapter 8! If you want your teen to come out on top, they need to have a positive mindset. And I'm not talking about just a "glass-half-full" attitude. I'm talking about the kind of mindset that makes them feel like they can conquer the world.

Teenagers face a multitude of challenges and pressures that have a significant impact on their mental health and subsequently, their perspective on life. As parents, we need to recognize the importance of nurturing a positive mentality in our teenagers and understand this plays a significant role in supporting their growth in this area.

So, gather 'round, folks, because in this chapter we aim to explore the significance of a positive mindset in teenagers, specifically focusing on its interconnected role with resilience and optimism. As my maternal grandfather Wayne used to say, "it's hard to see the roses properly while you're wearing shit colored glasses". Note; this was particularly funny because he was 100% blind almost his entire life.

We're exploring a way of thinking and perceiving the world that's rooted in optimism, resilience, and cultivating in our teenagers' a rock-solid belief in their ability to conquer any obstacle that comes their way. This isn't about slapping on a fake smile and pretending everything's peachy all the time. Heck no, it's about cultivating a psyche that transforms challenges into opportunities and garnering a dash of constructive optimism into their lives. And here's the cool part: science has our backs on this.

Research shows that a positive mindset boosts mental well-being, supercharges academic performance, nurtures healthy relationships, and amps up overall life satisfaction. So, let's make a toast to this remarkable mindset shift, because with a positive mentality in their arsenal, our teenagers can conquer the world.

Encouraging a positive mindset in your teen can help them in a multitude of ways. It helps them build resilience, develop healthy coping mechanisms, and boosts their self-esteem. A positive mindset also plays a pivotal role in nurturing healthy relationships, because teenagers with a positive ethos in life are more inclined to demonstrate empathy, kindness, and understanding towards others. Therefore, they can build strong and meaningful connections with their peers, family, and community, contributing to their overall social and emotional well-being. These positive relationships also provides them with a support network that can assist them in navigating difficult times as well as celebrating successes.

A positive mindset sets our stud muffin and stud muffinettes up for their future personal and professional lives, because as they transition into adulthood, they will encounter various challenges, such as career choices, academic pursuits, and personal goals. A positive attitude equips them with the mental resilience, self-belief, and problem-solving skills necessary to successfully navigate these challenges. It helps them develop a growth mindset, embrace challenges, and persist in the face of setbacks, continuously striving for self-improvement.

So how do you promote a positive mentality in your teen? First off, if you're constantly complaining and seeing the negative in situations, your teen is going to pick up on that. Instead, try to focus on the positives and find the silver lining in even the most difficult situations. When your teen sees you approach challenges with a positive attitude, they are more likely to adopt the same mindset. Uplift them to reframe negative thoughts into positive ones and focus on the good in any situation.

Another great way to instill positivity is through gratitude. Here's a nifty trick to fortify your teen's gratitude journey (more on this later) - have them whip out a daily gratitude list or keep a gratitude journal. I've been asking Noah what he is grateful for at least a few times per week since he learned to speak.

Your youngins, or anyone hanging around you long enough, will do as you do, not as you tell them to do. So, per usual... the crux of the matter, as always: lead by example. Express your own gratitude to others, and watch the magic happen. When your teen sees you showering appreciation on those who lend a helping hand or show kindness, they'll catch on and start dishing out their own gratitude-filled thank you's. It's a beautiful cycle.

Exploring The Link Between Mindset And Leadership

To grasp the significance of cultivating a positive mindset in leadership, it is necessary to delve into the concept of mindset itself and its impact on personal growth and leadership development. Mindset refers to a collection of beliefs, attitudes, and thoughts that shape how individuals perceive themselves and the world.

Mindset not only shapes how leaders view themselves, but also unleashes a tidal wave of inspiration and influence on those around them. Optimistic leaders are more likely to seek creative solutions and think outside the box when confronted with challenges. They approach problems with a positive attitude, focusing on discovering opportunities and possibilities rather than dwelling on limitations.

Plus, optimistic leaders are more prone to experience lower levels of stress, better manage their emotions, and maintain a positive work environment. They inspire and uplift their team members, inspire motivation, engagement, and overall job satisfaction.

A positive mindset fosters self-confidence. Leaders with a positive outlook believe in their abilities and possess a strong sense of self-assurance. They instill confidence in others, leading to increased trust and credibility within their team. If done well enough, this same quality will infectiously pass from their team to the outside world.

Optimistic leaders are more receptive to change and willing to explore new ideas and approaches. They embrace challenges as opportunities for growth and adjust their strategies accordingly. This adaptability enables leaders to navigate uncertain and rapidly changing environments, making them more effective in guiding their teams toward success.

By promoting a positive mindset in your teen, you are setting them up for success in all areas of their life. They will be better equipped to handle challenges, build strong relationships, and become effective and influential leaders.

Practical Steps For Cultivating A Positive Mindset In Your Teen

Let's take a closer look at some steps you can take to help cultivate a positive mindset in your teen:

1.   Promote Gratitude

Here's a tip for you, fellow parent: Help your teen find their groove and purpose in life. Inspire them to chase their passions and set meaningful goals. When they're on a mission that sets their soul on fire, they'll feel a sense of fulfillment and motivation like never before.

Let's not forget the beauty of both embracing challenges and making friends with mistakes, because mistakes are not monsters under the bed as most of us believe at one point or another in our early years; they're actually glorious opportunities for learning, growth and discovery. No one, ever, that did anything of any significance got there without making mistakes along the way. What better gift could one possibly bestow upon someone they love than granting them the ability to tackle challenges with a smile, knowing that every stumble is just a stepping stone to success. They'll become superheroes of resilience and conquerors of obstacles!

Now, here's a fun idea for you and your teen sidekick. How about starting a gratitude journal adventure? Each day, jot down three things you're both grateful for then share them. Noah and I do this before bedtime, or quite honestly, as many times as is necessary throughout the day. It could be as simple as savoring a mouthwatering meal, a spectacular sunset, or sharing a heartwarming conversation with a friend.

Sharing these notes at the end of the day or week adds some opportunities for light-heartedness and meaningful connection. If you want to go further there's a whole host of resources and ideas online to help.

2.   Challenge Negative Thoughts

Reframing negative thoughts is a powerful technique that can help your teen shift from a negative to a positive mindset. Spur them on to become aware of negative self-talk and challenge those thoughts with positive affirmations. For example, if your teen receives a poor grade on a test, they might think, "I'm not good enough and stupid and will never succeed." Help them challenge this thought by asking questions such as, "Is that really true?" or "What evidence do you have to support that thought?" Then ask the exact inverse "What about that statement is NOT true?" and "What evidence do you have to support that you ARE good enough?" Then, ask them to replace the negative thoughts with positive ones, such as, "I am capable and have many strengths." And "I may have struggled with this test, but I can work harder and improve." By practicing this technique, your teen can learn to shift their focus from negative to positive, leading to a more optimistic outlook on life.

3.   Create a Positive and Enriching Environment

Positive, supportive connections are like a shot of espresso for the soul. They lift us up, boost our self-esteem, and sprinkle some serious magic dust of well-being all around us. Some quick-fire ways to do this:

- Encourage open and honest communication among family members. Create an atmosphere where everyone feels comfortable expressing their thoughts, feelings, and concerns. Listen actively, show empathy, and validate each other's experiences.

- Healthy Boundaries: Establish healthy boundaries to ensure that each family member's needs and personal space are respected. Encourage open discussions about boundaries and consent, teaching family members to communicate their limits effectively.

- Quality Time and Fun Activities: Allocate regular quality time for family bonding. Engage in fun activities, such as game nights, outings, or shared hobbies. These experiences create positive memories, strengthen relationships, and enhance overall well-being.

- Conflict Resolution: Teach effective conflict resolution skills to manage disagreements constructively. Encourage family members to express their thoughts and feelings calmly and find mutually beneficial solutions. Foster a culture of forgiveness, understanding, and reconciliation.

4.   Model Positive Thinking

Modeling positive thinking is one of the most effective ways to motivate your teen to adopt a positive mindset. When they see you focusing on the good in situations and reframing challenges as opportunities for growth, they learn that positivity is a powerful tool for success. It's important to remember that your teen is always watching, and your attitude and behavior can significantly impact their mindset.

It is a major asset on this journey if you can learn to refrain from engaging in negative self-talk and criticism in the presence of your teen. Instead, Share your positive experiences and accomplishments with your teen, and encourage them to do the same. Demonstrate self-compassion and inspire your teenager to treat themselves kindly. By exemplifying positive thinking and self-compassion, you can support your teen in cultivating a more optimistic mindset and perspective on life.

A Story About John Mcavoy

John McAvoy, has a story that demonstrates the power of perseverance, transformation, and a positive mindset. John is currently a Nike athlete, however, he was previously a high profile armed robber who found redemption through the power of sport. Having broken both British and World records while in prison, he has embarked on a fresh journey as an endurance athlete and motivational speaker, dedicated to utilizing his rehabilitation journey to support and motivate others in transforming their lives positively.

His pivotal moment came when he found himself serving a second prison sentence. It was during this time that John experienced a profound change in perspective, when he learned of the passing of a close friend (due to crime) and began to question the world around him, his choices, and ultimately decided to turn his life around.

As he reflected on his choices and their consequences, John made a firm commitment to change his path. He discovered a passion for fitness and sports, specifically rowing and later triathlons. Believing that his past did not define his future, John embraced a positive mindset and focused on the transformative power of his journey.

With an unwavering determination and relentless work ethic, John gradually made progress. He trained relentlessly, pushing his physical and mental limits. He managed to set new British and World rowing records while in prison. The discipline required for his training also provided him with a sense of structure and purpose that he had longed for in his previous life.

Once out of prison, John's commitment paid off. He began competing in local races, steadily improving his performance. His dedication and positive mindset caught the attention of people within the triathlon community, who recognized his extraordinary transformation and resilience.

Despite facing financial hardships, John's unwavering belief in himself and his potential led him to achieve remarkable feats. He eventually qualified for professional races, competing against some of the world's top triathletes. His story resonated with people far beyond the triathlon community, inspiring others to overcome adversity and pursue their dreams.

Beyond his achievements in the triathlon world, John has become a motivational speaker, sharing his story of transformation and the power of a positive mindset. His experiences serve as a testament to the fact that our past does not define us and that we have the power to change our lives if we believe in ourselves.

John McAvoy's story is a testament to the resilience of the human spirit and the transformative power of a positive mindset. From a life of crime to becoming a celebrated triathlete, he demonstrates that with determination, dedication, and a belief in oneself, anyone can overcome their circumstances and create a better future. His journey serves as an inspiration to countless individuals, proving that even the most challenging paths can lead to extraordinary achievements.

Final Thoughts

In this chapter, we've delved into the important task of cultivating a kick-ass positive attitude in teenagers and how it ties to leadership. We've dug deep into the concept of mindset, the collection of beliefs, attitudes, and thoughts that shape how teenagers see themselves and the world.

So, why should we care about this positive mindset thing in leadership? Well, besides the fact that it actually impacts personal growth and leadership development, it can also help your teenager win friends and influence people (just ask Dale Carnegie!)

A positive mindset not only makes you feel warm and fuzzy inside, but it also enhances your problem-solving skills, leading you to creative solutions and alternative routes. With a positive mindset, challenges become opportunities for you to shine and show off your problem-solving prowess.

Developing leadership qualities can make you the life of the party. A positive mindset gives you the confidence to strut your stuff and believe in yourself. It's like having a secret stash of self-assurance that makes others go, "Dang, this person knows what they're doing!"

But, there's more to all this than just confidence. A positive mindset also turns you into a warrior of adaptability and flexibility, ready to tackle any challenge that comes your way.

And you're always up for trying new things. You become the champion of teamwork and collaboration, spreading good vibes and high-fives wherever you go. Who knew being a positive leader could turn you into an office rockstar?

Remember, we play a central role in this wild journey. We have the privilege to be the wise guides who show our kids the way and provide a nurturing environment for their positive mindset to flourish. With our support, they'll be ready to take on the world, armed with resilience, optimism, and a killer sense of humor.

Part 2 – Bring it to the World (external application)

Chapter 9: Buy your own car - Promoting Independence

As Mark Manson's Disappointment Panda says in his book The Subtle Art of Not Giving a F*ck: "Life is essentially an endless series of problems—the solution to one problem is merely the creation of the next. Don't hope for a life without problems. Hope for a life full of good problems."

The ultimate aim is to raise children who are self-reliant and capable of taking care of themselves. Yet, fostering independence in our teens can be a challenging task, particularly when they are still living under our roof. It's a delicate balance between providing support and nurturing, without crossing the line into over-protectiveness and solving all their problems for them. Life is full of obstacles and difficulties, and learning how to confront them, embrace them, make necessary changes, or even knowing when to walk away, is the only way to build resilience.

The Power Of Promoting Independence And Autonomy In Leadership

When it comes to being an effective leader, promoting independence is where it's at. Letting your team members fly solo, spread their wings, and do their thing not only makes them feel like badasses, but also unleashes their creativity and productivity. Just like setting a bunch of puppies loose in a room filled with chew toys and treats – they'll be bouncing off the walls with excitement and energy. And that's the kind of vibe you want in the workplace.

When you advocate independence, you're basically saying to your team members, "Hey, I trust you. You got this." And that kind of validation is like a pat on the back from Chuck Norris himself. It shows that you respect their abilities and believe in their potential. And let's be honest, who doesn't love a little bit of recognition and respect?

Promoting independence doesn't just benefit teams, it helps leaders too. By giving team members the freedom to do their own thing, you tap into a varied range of skills and approaches that you never knew existed, or a delicious feast of new ideas and solutions, if you will. And that's the kind of innovation that takes your organization from "meh" to "wow" The sky's the limit! Or, you know, the ceiling. But still, it's pretty darn impressive.

Independence Day! Encouraging Independence In Your Teen

Promoting independence in teenage children can indeed be a complex endeavor. We have a few tricks up our sleeves to make the journey more manageable and enjoyable. With some (tongue-in-cheek) dialogues to engage your teen's decision-making skills, we'll explore effective methods to foster self-sufficiency and enhance their confidence.

1. It's your call, kid: Allow them to make their own decisions

We looked at effective decision making in Chapter 4, and it's one of the most important ways to promote independence in our teens. For now, forget the wonderfully insightful and practical points for you and your teenager to read over with a fine-tooth comb, here's a lighthearted example of what you can say:

"Well son/daughter, you know what they say - give a teenager a fish and you feed them for a day, but teach a teenager to fish, and you feed them for a lifetime. And that's what we're doing here. By letting you choose your own clothes, pick your own activities, and even decide on your own meals, I'm helping you learn how to make good decisions. Plus, it saves me the hassle of having to figure out what to make for dinner every night."

2.   Teach them life skills

"Well kiddo, you may not believe it, but one day you'll be out in the big, wide world all on your own. And when that day comes, you'll want to be ready. That's why we're teaching you these life skills now - cooking, cleaning, laundry, basic home repairs... all the things you need to know to be a self-sufficient, independent adult. And who knows, maybe someday you'll even thank me when you're the only one in your dorm who knows how to unclog a toilet or snake a drain!"

Another way to promote independence is by teaching our teens life skills that will help them become more self-sufficient. This includes skills like cooking, cleaning, laundry, and basic home repairs. By teaching them these skills, we are giving them the tools they need to take care of themselves once they leave home.

3.   Uplift them to help them take on responsibilities

Now, listen up, we should instill a sense of responsibility in our teenage offspring, not only within the confines of our humble abodes but also in their community. One way to do this is by encouraging them to take on tasks such as babysitting younger siblings, lending a helping hand at a local charity, or even working part-time. By doing so, we help our teens become more accountable and self-sufficient, and they gain valuable skills that will serve them well in their future endeavors. You can phrase your skit to your teen something like this:

"Well son/daughter, you know what they say - with great power comes great responsibility. And now that you're getting older, it's time for you to start taking on some of that responsibility. Whether it's helping out with your younger siblings, volunteering at a charity, or even getting a part-time job, you're learning some valuable life lessons. You'll learn the importance of hard work, accountability, and making a difference in your community. And who knows, maybe someday you'll be the boss of your own company, with a whole team of people looking up to you for guidance and leadership! You don't want to mess that up, now, do you?!"

Letting our teens take on responsibilities is like giving them a big ol' dose of confidence juice! Mmm.. juice. Remember that whole "Confidence breeds confidence" thing? While creating competence in their capacity to care for themselves, more likely than not, they will gain a whole new perspective on life. Plus, it's the perfect opportunity for them to flex their empathy muscles and learn how to work well with others. And, let's not forget about the power of positive reinforcement - who doesn't love a good pat on the back for a job well done? So go ahead and support your teen to take on some responsibility. They might, probably darn well will, surprise you (and themselves) with what they're capable of!

4.   Don't be a space invader: Give them space

As parents, we sometimes tend to micromanage our kids' lives, like a pesky fly that won't buzz off. But we need to realize that our teens need space to spread their wings and fly. Giving them the freedom to socialize with their friends, dive into their hobbies and passions, and explore their curiosities is like giving them a breath of fresh air. It shows them that we trust them and respect their choices while also giving them a chance to become independent individuals.

Here's how that particular convo could go down:

"Well son/daughter, I know I love spending time with you, but I also know that it's important for you to spread your wings a little bit. You're becoming your own person, with your own interests, hobbies, and friends. And that's great! (By God, it's been a long time coming!) It's important for you to have the space and freedom to explore those things without me constantly hovering over you. You're a responsible young adult, and I trust you to make good decisions. So go out there and have some fun, make some memories, and don't forget to come back home and tell me all about it!"

Noah's Journey To Independence

When my son Noah turned 14, he started to express a desire for more independence. At first, I was hesitant to give him too much freedom, but I realized that it was necessary for him to start learning how to take care of himself. I encouraged him to take on more responsibilities at home, like doing his own laundry and cooking his own meals.

One day, Noah approached me with a proposition. He wanted to start cooking dinner for the family (him and I) once a week. I was hesitant initially, but I eventually agreed to let him try it. He spent hours planning the menu, going grocery shopping, and preparing the meal. When it was finally ready, we sat down to eat, and I have to say, not only was it one of the better meals we've shared together watching him beam with pride, but his appreciation level for when I make him food increased tremendously.

From then on, Noah took over cooking duties once a week, and eventually started helping out with other household tasks like cleaning and grocery shopping. He also started taking on more responsibilities outside of the home, like working part-time at our BJJ school (shout out to Eidson Jiu Jitsu).

Watching Noah become more independent and self-sufficient has been one of the greatest joys of my life. While it wasn't always easy to give him the space he needed, it was worth it to see him grow into the responsible, confident young man he is today.

Inspiring Reflections On Nurturing Independence

We all know that our teens will eventually grow up and become independent beings who think they know everything. But as we learned, encouraging independence is actually a good thing. It helps teenagers develop pivotal life skills and prepares them to conquer the world.

Finding the right balance is key. We want our teens to spread their wings and fly, but we also want to keep them from crashing and burning. As we dove into the practical steps for promoting independence, we covered ground on the importance of giving our kids the space to make decisions, even if they stumble and fall along the way. After all, who doesn't love a good face plant? But seriously, we'll be there, as always to support them, whether it's to weigh the pros and cons by creating a list, discussing possible outcomes, or for them to seek our advice when needed (aka, a quick Google search).

Promoting independence doesn't mean abandoning our teenagers in the wilderness. Nope, it means being there as their safety net and their guiding light when the darkness gets a bit too overwhelming.

In the end, promoting independence in teenagers is all about preparing them for the chaos of the real world. We want them to learn, grow, and become their own heroes. So, embrace the chaos, and guide your teenager to unleash their independence in the most epic and hilarious ways possible. Because life is too short to be boring, and our teenagers deserve to conquer the world with style and a dash of mischief.

Chapter 10: Teaching Time Management

In today's fast-paced world, time management has become a vital skill for success. Most parents wish we had more hours in a day to get everything done – I mean, who doesn't as an adult? By guiding our teens to understand the benefits of effective time management skills we can help them succeed in their academic and personal pursuits and give them this skill early in life. We will look at ways to provide them with this fundamental skill that will help them stay organized, prioritize their tasks, reduce stress, and accomplish their goals, leading to more efficient and productive use of their time.

Forget about obsessing over productivity hacks or ticking off tasks on a checklist (I addressed this in great detail in The Lazy Person's Guide to Productivity and Outsmart Overthinking) mastering the art of time management runs deeper than that and helps our teens unlock a whole new level of productivity and make their decisions faster than Neo dodges bullets in The Matrix. When your teen can manage their time effectively, they become assured, relaxed, and a master of their destiny. They'll have the power to tackle challenges head-on, meet deadlines like a time-traveling wizard, and juggle multiple tasks without breaking a sweat.

Not to mention, that we shouldn't overlook the stress-busting benefits of effective time management. Say goodbye to watching those sleepless nights and panicked cramming sessions. With proper time management, they'll have the mental space to breathe, relax, and even enjoy the occasional meme break. Your teen's brain will thank you for that!

Why is time management so fundamental in leadership and for teenagers? Well, unostentatiously, time is your (our) most precious resource. It's even more valuable than the latest gaming console or a lifetime supply of pizza (although your teen may highly disagree). So, let's get into it.

Why Is Time Management Important For Leadership?

Let's have a discussion on the captivating realm of time management and its profound significance in leadership. That might sound sarcastic, but genuinely, I can attest to the importance of the subject, so let's unravel the intricate connection between effective time management, goal achievement, and success.

Time management is the ultimate power-up for a successful leader, like having a Mario star that lets you run through walls of distractions, procrastination, and wasted time. In the realm of leadership, the ability to manage time effectively becomes a necessity, enabling leaders to navigate the complex landscape of tasks, priorities, and deadlines.

Leaders who master the art of time management exude a sense of discipline, focus, and efficiency. They are adept at juggling a multitude of responsibilities, allocating time wisely, and making the most of every moment. This mastery enhances their leadership effectiveness, as they inspire others through their ability to lead by example and accomplish tasks with precision and timeliness.

Furthermore, time management fosters accountability and strategic thinking. When leaders manage their time effectively, they become accountable for their time and actions, setting a powerful example for their team. Strategic thinking blossoms as leaders gain the mental space to reflect, plan, and make informed decisions. By optimizing their time, leaders unlock their strategic prowess and guide their teams toward success with clarity and purpose.

Mastering The Time Game: Instilling Time Management Skills In Your Teen

One of the first steps in fostering time management skills is to help our teens understand the importance of prioritizing tasks. Support your teen to make a list of tasks and prioritize them based on their urgency and importance. This will help them focus on the most critical tasks first, and avoid wasting time on less important ones.

There are many effective ways to prioritize tasks. Here are a few great strategies:

1. Make a to-do list: This may seem obvious, but making a to-do list is a great way to prioritize tasks. Write down everything you need to do, and then rank them in order of importance. Usually, just getting it out in front of you will relieve a bit of the stress before the list is even organized. You can use a paper planner (I have a Time Mastery Planner on Amazon for just this), a digital task manager, or any other tool that works for you.

2. Use the ABCD method: This method involves labeling tasks as either A, B, C, or D. A tasks are the most important, B tasks are important but not urgent, C tasks are nice to do but not urgent, and D tasks can be delegated or eliminated. Focus on completing all of the A tasks first, then move on to the B tasks, and so on.

3. Consider urgency and importance: Another effective way to prioritize tasks is to consider both urgency and importance. Urgent tasks require immediate attention, while important tasks contribute to your long-term goals. By prioritizing both urgency and importance, you can tackle tasks in a way that makes the most sense for your overall goals.

4. Use the Eisenhower Matrix: The Eisenhower Matrix, also known as the Eisenhower Decision Matrix, is a time management tool that helps individuals prioritize tasks based on their urgency and importance. It is named after Dwight D. Eisenhower, the 34th

President of the United States, who was known for his effective time management skills.

The matrix is divided into four quadrants, formed by two axes representing urgency and importance:

1. Urgent and Important: Tasks in this quadrant are both urgent and important, requiring immediate attention. They usually involve critical deadlines, important projects, or crises. These tasks should be tackled first and given high priority.

2. Important but Not Urgent: Tasks in this quadrant are important but not time-sensitive. They contribute to long-term goals, personal growth, and strategic planning. Examples include relationship building, skill development, and goal setting. These tasks should be scheduled and given dedicated time to ensure they are not overlooked.

3. Urgent but Not Important: Tasks in this quadrant are urgent but don't have significant long-term impact. They often include interruptions, distractions, or activities that can be delegated. It's important to minimize or eliminate these tasks as much as possible to free up time for more important activities.

4. Not Urgent and Not Important: Tasks in this quadrant are neither urgent nor important. They are time-wasters, trivial activities, or distractions that don't contribute to personal or professional goals. It's advisable to eliminate or delegate these tasks whenever possible to focus on more meaningful activities.

By using the Eisenhower Matrix, individuals can effectively prioritize their tasks, manage their time, and avoid getting overwhelmed by urgent but unimportant activities. It helps in maintaining focus on tasks that align with long-term goals and lead to personal and professional success.

No one wants a teenager that's stressed out and always rushing around, or running late. It's chaos. The first step is to elicit different methods until they find the one that suits them best. The best way to prioritize tasks will depend on the nature of the tasks themselves. Your teen should also remember to take a breather and recharge their batteries with a walk, some physical activity, or even a nice hot cup of tea. And here are some other key areas to reflect on and implement with your teenager to help them stay on track.

Use Clear Goals and Priorities: In Chapter 6, we looked at the SMART framework for creating goals, if you need to, go back and refamiliarize yourself, and your teen, with this framework. By setting clear goals, breaking down the necessary step to achieve them, and understanding what problems and pitfalls we might encounter we can plan our time and schedules accordingly to factor in what we need to do and the time each task requires.

Planning and Organizing: Motivate your teen to use a planner to keep track of their schedule, assignments, and deadlines. They can use a physical or digital planner, whichever they prefer. Encourage your teen to create a schedule to manage their time. This can help them see what tasks need to be accomplished and when. Note: This is also helpful when categorizing their to do list. They can break down their day into blocks of time for schoolwork, extracurricular activities, chores, and leisure time. You can also introduce them to an arsenal of time management tools and techniques, from digital to-do lists and calendars to apps that transform scattered thoughts into structured schedules. The world of Ai is having a significant impact on the way we work and stay organized. Apps such as Notion can be invaluable to your teen. I recommend checking it out.

Developing Effective Time-Tracking Strategies: Become their time-tracking guru as you guide teenagers on a journey of self-awareness. Galvanize them to' don their detective hats, and observe how they spend their precious minutes, there are loads of apps to help with this and smart phones have these insights built in. With newfound insights, they'll uncover hidden time thieves and you can even encourage them to set a daily time limit for the worst offending apps.

Practicing Self-Discipline And Avoiding Procrastination:

Time management also involves the ability to say no to distractions. Reinforce to your teen to limit their time on social media, video games, or other non-productive activities. Instead, help them find ways to incorporate breaks and relaxation into their schedule, so they can recharge and stay focused while remaining structured.

A Further Note On Overcoming Procrastination

Ah, the sweet allure of procrastination. Why do today what you can do tomorrow, right? Well, as tempting as that may be, it's not the best approach to time management, obviously. We all know that, but yet, still it somehow persists in rearing its ugly head. So, how can we help our teens tackle their to-do lists without getting overwhelmed?

One key strategy is to break down larger tasks into smaller, more manageable ones. It's like eating an elephant one bite at a time as my Hungarian grandfather used to say (not that we condone that sort of thing). You can't do it all at once, but if you take it one bite at a time, eventually, you'll finish the whole thing.

Support your teen to set realistic goals and deadlines for each step. And I'm not talking about "finish the entire project by tomorrow at noon." That's a recipe for disaster. Overwhelmed disaster at that. Instead, set smaller goals that are achievable within a specific timeframe. For example, "research for 30 minutes today" or "write 500 words by the end of the week." By breaking the larger task into smaller chunks, it becomes less daunting and more manageable.

Let's also not forget about the power of deadlines. Without them, tasks can linger on indefinitely, but with a deadline, there's a sense of urgency and a greater likelihood of getting things done. Just make sure the deadlines are realistic and achievable. Otherwise, your teen may end up feeling even more overwhelmed and stressed when their tasks are all laid out.

So, to sum it up: experiment to see what works, help them to prioritize tasks, break down larger tasks into manageable chunks, set realistic goals and deadlines, and avoid the temptation of procrastination. Your teen will be well on their way to becoming a time-management master, in, err.. no time.

Here are some additional tips that can help lighten the load for your teenager as

they learn time management:

1. Time blocking: Motivate your teenager to allocate dedicated time slots for various activities like studying, exercising, socializing, and leisure. This fosters a structured schedule and guarantees appropriate focus on each task. When they are studying the pomodoro technique which help block productivity into chunk of 25 minutes with 5 minutes break and then a longer break after each hour is a great way to help them structure their time.

2. Avoid multitasking: Advise your teenager to concentrate on one task at a time instead of attempting to handle multiple tasks simultaneously. This approach helps prevent distractions and enhances productivity.

3. Take breaks: Suggest to your teenager the importance of incorporating regular breaks into their study or

work sessions. Taking brief intervals can actually boost productivity and guard against burnout.

4. Be flexible: Teach your teen to be flexible with their time management, as unexpected events and interruptions can happen. Encourage them to adjust their schedule as needed while still staying focused on their goals.

5. Minimize distractions: Distractions can significantly consume time. Motivate your teenager to reduce distractions by disabling their phone notification temporarily while focusing on a task. I actually have my notifications muted permanently on my device so I can exercise agency in what I am intentionally giving my attention to opposed to being reflexively pulled in multiple disruptive directions. Additionally, they can seek a tranquil environment to work without interruptions.

A Story About Noah

Let's talk about Noah, as a middle schooler my son knew the struggle of poor time management all too well. He was always cramming for tests and burning the midnight oil to finish his assignments around a busy schedule that included a lot of activities he loved doing, such as BJJ. Poor guy was probably more tired than a sloth on a Monday morning (do sloths work on a Monday morning? Or at all for that matter? I doubt it. Too busy crossing roads slowly, damn, maybe that IS their job! Who knew.) Anyway, when I recognized this, I stepped in to help him find strategies to help him, including those discussed in this chapter, and he started to turn things around by creating a schedule and prioritizing his tasks.

He learned to break down larger assignments into smaller, more manageable tasks, and set deadlines for himself. He even turned off his phone while studying to avoid distractions - now that's some self-control right there! These time management skills helped Noah improve his grades and become calmer and happier as his stress and anxiety levels reduced. A beautiful side benefit he actually brought up with me was that it took him significantly less time to complete his homework (which obviously wasn't his favorite task).

Noah also became more confident in his ability to manage his time effectively and developed an awareness of what he could and couldn't commit to, and achieve, in an allotted timeframe. He continued to implement these skills throughout his academic and personal life. I have to say, I am super proud of how organized, efficient, and relaxed he is these days. His success is a prime example of how effective time management skills can positively impact a teen's confidence, academic life, and approach to their personal endeavors.

Without these skills, students can feel as lost as Gollum without his precious. They may become overwhelmed and stressed, leading to a decline in their academic performance and overall well-being. But by creating a schedule and breaking down larger tasks into smaller, more manageable ones, students like Noah can prioritize their workload and use their time more efficiently. Setting deadlines for themselves also helps them stay on track and avoid procrastination.

And let's not overlook minimizing distractions like social media. This was a game-changer for Noah. It's like Thanos snapping his fingers and erasing a mind-bending quantity of distractions from existence - poof, they're gone!

We can all help set our kids up for success in their academic and personal pursuits by teaching them the art of time management. And, of course, as always, it's important to lead by example to help our teens develop this art.

The Time Warrior's Wisdom: Teaching Time Management To Teenagers

As we reach the culmination of our time management expedition, it is vital to reflect on the profound significance of this skill in shaping leadership qualities in our teens. Time management, like a trusted compass, guides them on a path toward leadership success, enabling them to navigate the complexities of their responsibilities effectively, and not be that one kid who's ALWAYS late.

Beyond the immediate benefits of productivity and reduced stress, effective time management plants the seeds of personal growth and cultivates a harmonious work-life balance. By mastering the art of allocating time wisely, teenagers unlock the door to self-discovery, self-discipline, and the fulfillment of their aspirations.

Recognizing time as a valuable currency, investing it astutely and guarding against its reckless squandering, are wise approaches. By embracing lifelong time management, teenagers (and adults) empower themselves to achieve goals, unlock their inherent potential, and leave a lasting impact on the world.

Who knows, maybe your teenager will become the next Jobs, Musk or Bezos, and lead the charge toward a brighter future. Empowered greatly by their mastering of the art of time management.

Chapter 11: The Mentorship Quest

Welcome to Chapter 11. Let's dive into the world of mentors and how they can shape our teen's path to leadership greatness.

Imagine this: you're a young teenager, and you've got dreams, aspirations, a boatload of energy, and maybe a little bit of confusion. You've got all these ideas swirling around in your head, but you're not exactly sure how to bring them to life. Enter mentors as wise and experienced guides.

"If I have seen further, it is by standing on the shoulders of giants."

~ Isaac Newton wrote in a 1675 letter to fellow scientist Robert Hooke.

See, in the end, I did check that quote, and I was right, it wasn't Mark Twain! Mentors bring a treasure trove of experience that will take your teen's development and leadership game to the next level. Mentors have been there, done that, and probably have the T-shirt to prove it (or maybe a cool mug with an inspirational quote, who knows?). They have battle scars, war stories, and nuggets of wisdom that'll blow your teenager's mind.

Beyond their wisdom, mentors can be the ultimate GPS navigation systems to help our young teens navigate through the twists and turns of development, mindset, and leadership. They guide them through the treacherous paths of leadership - like those friendly voices in your car telling you to take a U-turn when you're about to drive off a cliff. We all need that, trust me.

A good, supportive mentor will be a strong advocate and source of encouragement for your teenager, offering guidance and support throughout their journey. When our teens stumble and fall (which they will, because we all do), mentors are there with open arms to help pick them up, dust them off, and give them a motivational speech that would make even Rocky Balboa shed a tear! Mentors are another person and another voice to help uplift our teens at their darkest hour and one more person who has their back. Think about that for a moment. Its value is incalculable. Mentors help make your teen believe in themselves even on their toughest days.

While we're on the topic, motivational speeches! Have you ever seen Israel Adesanya's inspirational speech after his UFC 287 victory over Alex Pereira? It doesn't get much more motivational than this:

After suffering a stunning knockout defeat at the hands of Alex Pereira in November 2022, Adesanya bounced back in a big way to stop Pereira in their rematch on a Saturday night (April 8th, 2023) in Miami.

Adesanya, who suffered his first defeat at 185 pounds when Pereira scored the late fifth-round finish at UFC 281, felt the weight of the world on him in the weeks and months that followed. The New Zealand resident said he used all that as motivation to come back and reclaim his title.

Adesanya took the microphone from UFC announcer Joe Rogan before he could even ask him a question to deliver quite the speech on overcoming adversity.

"I need to say something. Listen to me. I hope every one of you behind the screens in this arena can feel this level of happiness just one time in your life. I hope all of you can feel how f---ing happy I am just once in your life, But guess what? You will never feel this level of happiness if you don't go for something in your own life. When they knock you down, when they try and shit on you, when they talk shit about you, and they try and put their foot on your neck, if you stay down, you will never get that resolve. Fortify your mind and feel this level of happiness one time in your life. I'm blessed to be able to feel this shit again and again and again and again and again."

Wow! Adesanya's sheer joy in the aftermath of the win was a sight to behold. The depth of joy that only comes from something you have poured your heart and soul into. Something you have worked tirelessly and passionately toward. A mission that you can blindly commit to because you trust your coaches, mentors, leaders, trainers, teammates, and yourself. They say you become who you hang around... he MUST have some pretty incredible people he trusts to guide him to elicit that degree of commitment and, therefore, reward.

Let's circle back to Mentors then because they also bring a secret weapon to the table: inspiration. They're like these walking, talking, living examples of what young teens can become. They ignite that fire within, fueling their passion and pushing them to reach for a whole new level of what is possible.

Guiding Lights: The Hidden Power Of Mentorship In Leadership

Within the domain of the leadership ladder, the importance of seeking mentors cannot be overstated. Mentors serve as guiding lights, illuminating the path to personal and professional growth. With their wealth of experience and wisdom, they offer a unique perspective that can help aspiring leaders navigate challenges, hone essential skills, and unlock their true potential.

Learning from someone who has already traversed the terrain is paramount in leadership. By tapping into their invaluable insights, aspiring leaders can learn from their mentors' triumphs and tribulations, gaining practical wisdom and avoiding the common pitfalls that lie in wait. Mentors provide more than just advice; they share real-life stories, offer constructive feedback, and nurture decision-making prowess, enabling individuals to make more informed choices on their leadership journey.

Beyond knowledge transfer, their success stories resonate with anyone aspiring to follow in their footsteps by illuminating what is possible with dedication and perseverance. Witnessing a mentor's accomplishments and hearing their tales of resilience instills confidence. In the presence of a mentor who believes in their potential, mentees are emboldened to step out of their comfort zones, embrace growth opportunities, and borrow the sense of certainty required to reach for greatness.

It's not only about personal growth either, no, it's also about unlocking a world of connections and networking. A good mentor has a network that would make a social media influencer jealous, all cultivated through years of blood, sweat, and achievement within their field. By forging connections through mentorship, aspiring leaders gain access to influential individuals within their industry, creating a ripple effect of opportunities and collaborations with other seasoned professionals. Building relationships in this way propels individuals forward, fast-tracking their leadership journey.

Mentors also provide ongoing support and guidance. They serve as trusted allies, offering a listening ear and objective perspectives. Mentors help mentees examine situations from fresh angles, fostering critical thinking and personal growth. Beyond formal discussions, mentors genuinely care about their mentees' well-being, offering encouragement during challenging times and celebrating achievements. It is through these enduring connections that mentorship blossoms into a transformative force in leadership.

Unlocking the Power of Mentorship: Building Leadership Skills for the Future

Mentorship can be a boost of courage that helps our teens step into their power and believe in themselves more than they otherwise would. With the guidance and support of a mentor, our teens can conquer their self-doubt and embrace their unique abilities. They'll walk taller, speak louder, and radiate that confidence that will inspire others to follow their lead. This can profoundly influence your teen, not just in the immediate years but throughout their lives.

Research shows that youth mentoring by non-parent adults, models positive social skills and facilitates interpersonal connections beyond family, helps teens interpret and manage life challenges, including relationships with peers and parents, and strengthens self-regulation and their ability to manage emotions, and think before acting.

Mentors challenge teenagers to step out of their comfort zones, explore their strengths, and confront their weaknesses. When it comes to personal growth and self-awareness, mentorship is a mirror that reflects their true potential and areas for improvement. Mentors are like that super cool professor who teaches real-life lessons that textbooks can't capture. They pass on their wisdom, expertise, and practical know-how, equipping our kids with the tools they need to navigate the world of leadership. Through this journey of self-discovery, our teens develop a deep understanding of who they are and what they stand for.

Here are some key reasons why mentors are so important in nurturing the potential of your teenager:

1. Experience and Expertise: Mentors bring valuable experience and expertise to the table. They have likely faced similar challenges and obstacles in their own leadership journeys and can offer insights on how to navigate them effectively. Their knowledge and expertise can help teenagers avoid common pitfalls and make informed decisions, setting them on a path to success.

2. Role Models and Inspiration: Having a mentor allows teenagers to have someone to look up to and emulate. Mentors serve as positive role models exemplifying the qualities and skills necessary for effective leadership. By observing and learning from their mentors, teenagers can develop a clear vision of the kind of leader they want to be and gain inspiration to achieve their goals.

3. Personalized Guidance: Mentors provide personalized guidance tailored to the specific needs and goals of the teenage leader. They take the time to understand the teenager's strengths, weaknesses, and aspirations and provide tailored advice and support. This personalized approach helps teenagers develop their unique leadership style and capitalize on their strengths while working on areas that need improvement.

4. Emotional Support and Empowerment: Life's journey can be challenging and, at times, overwhelming for teenagers. Mentors provide much-needed support, encouragement, motivation, and a listening ear. They help teenagers build resilience, overcome self-doubt, and develop a positive mindset that is imperative for effective leadership. Mentors empower teenagers to believe in themselves and their abilities, enabling them to overcome obstacles and reach their full potential.

5. Networking and Connections: Mentors often have a wide network of contacts and connections in various fields. They can introduce teenagers to influential people, opportunities, and resources that can accelerate their growth and expand their horizons. Mentors can open doors for teenagers, connecting them with relevant professionals, organizations, or platforms that can further their leadership development.

6. Constructive Feedback and Accountability: One of the most valuable aspects of mentorship is the opportunity for constructive feedback. Mentors provide objective insights, highlighting areas of improvement and offering suggestions for growth. This feedback helps teenagers gain self-awareness, develop critical skills, and refine their leadership abilities. Mentors also hold teenagers accountable for their actions and goals, ensuring they stay focused and committed to their leadership development.

Let's look at setting the stage for the quest of finding mentors with our teenagers. When we set the stage for seeking mentors, we're equipping these young minds with a mindset that's hungry for mentorship. They understand the value of having a guiding hand, like a compass pointing them in the right direction. They know that mentors are like Sherpas on Mount Everest, ready to help them conquer their leadership peaks.

By understanding their goals and needs, our teens know exactly what they're looking for in a mentor. And they actively seek out these mentors. They don't wait for mentors to magically appear in their lives. No, they'll take charge, go out there, and find mentors who will shape their leadership destiny.

Here are some key aspects to consider when setting the stage for seeking proper mentors:

• Awareness of the Benefits: Create awareness with your teenager and educate them about how mentors can provide guidance, support, and wisdom, and how this can positively impact their life and leadership journey. Highlight real-life examples of successful mentorship stories to illustrate the transformative power of mentors.

• Encouraging Openness and Willingness: Create an environment that fosters openness and willingness to seek mentorship. Help your teenager understand that seeking guidance and support is a sign of strength and a valuable opportunity for growth. Uplift them to embrace the idea of learning from others and being receptive to different perspectives. Emphasize the importance of humility and a growth mindset in the mentorship process.

• Providing Mentorship Resources: Equip your teen (and yourself) with resources to facilitate the mentorship search. Here are some areas for you to explore:

o Nonprofit Organizations: Numerous nonprofit organizations offer mentorship programs specifically designed for teenagers. Examples include Big Brothers Big Sisters, Boys & Girls Clubs of America, and Junior Achievement. These organizations aim to match young individuals with mentors who can provide guidance and support.

o Local Community Organizations: Explore community centers, libraries, or youth organizations in your area. They may offer mentorship programs or be aware of individuals willing to mentor teenagers in specific fields or interests.

o Online Platforms: Utilize online platforms that connect mentors with mentees. Websites like Youth.gov, Mentoring.org, and Spark Teen offer virtual mentorship opportunities for teenagers. These platforms often have mentors from various backgrounds and fields who can provide guidance remotely.

o Professional Associations: Investigate professional associations related to your interests, such as science, arts, sports, or technology. Some associations have mentorship programs or resources available for young individuals looking to learn from professionals in the field.

o   Alumni Networks: If you have a particular interest in a college or university, reach out to their alumni network. Alumni from your desired institution may be willing to mentor teenagers and provide insights into their career paths and experiences.

o   Personal Connections: Don't overlook the power of personal connections. Seek out family friends, relatives, or acquaintances who have experience or knowledge in fields you're interested in. They might be willing to mentor and guide you through their insights and expertise.

• Cultivating a Mentorship Mindset: Foster a mentorship mindset by emphasizing the value of learning from others and the willingness to seek guidance. Motivate your teen to reflect on their own strengths and areas for growth and how mentorship can contribute to their personal development. Instilling a mentorship mindset early on helps teenagers understand the importance of seeking mentors as an ongoing practice throughout their leadership journey.

• Parental Support and Involvement: Parents and guardians play a vital role in setting the stage for seeking mentors. They can support and guide teenagers in identifying their goals, provide encouragement and support throughout the mentorship process, and assist with making initial connections. You can also advocate for your teen by leveraging your networks to help find suitable mentors.

Nurturing Mentor-Mentee Connections: Unleashing The Power Of Guidance

A good place to start with mentor-finding is by identifying your beloved teenager's specific needs and goals. Understanding what makes their heart race and their mind tingle is key to finding a mentor match. Take the time to sit down with them, ask them questions, and really listen to their dreams and aspirations. Do they want to conquer the world of technology or dive into the depths of art? Knowing their unique needs and goals will serve you both well on this journey.

With a clear picture of what your teenager is after, it's time to define the desired qualities and expertise in a mentor. Are they looking for someone with a wealth of experience in their chosen field? Or maybe they want a mentor who can ignite their creative spark and push them out of their comfort zone? Get specific. Create a mentor wishlist, and put it into action.

Tap into existing networks and communities. This is where the power of connections comes into play. Look around, and you'll realize that you're surrounded by a potential mentor gold mine. Friends, family, teachers, coaches, local organizations - they all have the potential to be the bridge between your teenager and their mentor match. Don't underestimate the power of these networks and communities. They can be the secret to unlocking mentorship opportunities. So, put on your thinking hat and start exploring the hidden gems right before you.

It's time for your teen to put those communication skills to work and reach out to potential mentors. This may sound daunting to your teenager, but help them see the benefits of the right way to do this, like approaching a cool, wise stranger at a party. Craft a thoughtful message or make a simple phone call expressing your teenager's admiration and interest in their expertise. Be authentic. Help them to let their passion and excitement shine through. Remember, mentors are often flattered by the opportunity to share their knowledge and make a difference in someone's life. So, tell them to take a deep breath and press that send button.

Cultivating a mutually beneficial relationship with a mentor takes time, care, and a sprinkle of patience. Motivate your teenager to be proactive in their engagement with their mentor. Support them to come prepared with questions, to seek feedback, and to be open to new perspectives. Remind them that mentorship is a two-way street where both parties can learn and grow together. It's a dance of mutual respect and support. Water that mentorship plant and watch it bloom into something truly remarkable.

There will be challenges and setbacks, but as we've already covered resilience in Chapter 6, you know what to do. Remind your teenager that setbacks are not roadblocks but opportunities for growth. Fortify them to stay persistent, to adapt their approach if needed, and to keep their eyes on the prize. The perfect mentor is out there, waiting to be found.

A Story About Elon

Many of us have heard of Elon Musk, the visionary entrepreneur and founder of companies like Tesla, SpaceX, and Neuralink.

Throughout his career, Musk has sought out mentors who have played a significant role in shaping his entrepreneurial journey. One notable mentor in Musk's life is James R. Cantrell, a renowned aerospace engineer and entrepreneur. Cantrell became a mentor to Musk during his early ventures, offering guidance and expertise in the field of rocketry. Their collaboration led to the founding of SpaceX, a groundbreaking private space exploration company that has revolutionized the aerospace industry.

Another influential mentor in Musk's life is Larry Page, the co-founder of Google. Page provided valuable guidance and insights to Musk, particularly in the realms of technology and innovation. Their mentor-mentee relationship allowed Musk to gain a deeper understanding of the digital landscape and inspired him to pursue ambitious projects, such as the development of electric vehicles and sustainable energy solutions through Tesla.

Additionally, Musk credits Robert Zubrin, an aerospace engineer and advocate for Mars exploration, as a mentor who influenced his vision for space exploration and the colonization of Mars. Zubrin's mentorship helped shape

Musk's long-term goal of making humanity a multi-planetary species, as evidenced by SpaceX's ambitious plans for interplanetary travel.

By seeking out mentors with expertise in various fields, Musk was able to leverage their knowledge and guidance to accelerate his entrepreneurial endeavors. The mentorship he received provided him with the necessary insights, industry connections, and support to overcome challenges and achieve groundbreaking success.

Musk's story underscores the transformative power of mentorship in the realm of entrepreneurship. Through the mentorship of Cantrell, Page, Zubrin, and others, he was able to combine their wisdom with his own vision and drive to revolutionize industries and advance human progress. Musk's journey serves as a reminder of the immense value that mentors can bring to one's life, offering guidance, inspiration, and a wealth of experience that can propel individuals toward achieving extraordinary goals.

Final Thoughts On Seeking Mentors

By now (if you've been paying attention!), you'll have a good idea of how to cook up the sauce that transforms your teen into a rock star of greatness. Mentorship is a big deal. With a mentor by their side, our kids can conquer self-doubt and unleash their inner confidence.

Personal growth is where our teens can shed their old skin and step into their true potential. It's like that moment when you finally embrace your weirdness and say, "Hell yeah, this is me!" They're like the wise sages passing on ancient wisdom, but instead of long white beards, they've got stylish haircuts and probably a Spotify playlist of motivational jams. A great mentor can be a buddy who calls you out on your BS and says, "Dude, get your act together!" It's a loving kick up the backside, if you will.

Let's raise our metaphorical glasses to the power of mentorship. Embrace it, nurture it, and watch our young leaders soar to new heights of greatness. Now, go forth and spread the mentorship love. The revolution begins now!

Chapter 12: Teamwork Makes the Dream Work: Encouraging Collaboration

Emphasizing the power of collaboration is a cool concept to work on with your teen. We're encouraging no more lone wolves and helping them see the benefits of working with others. In today's world, where everything is all about "team effort," the ability to collaborate is more valuable than ever. In short, we need team players. So, instead of letting your teen lock themselves away in their room, propel them to get out there and work with others. They can start by joining a club (I highly recommend BJJ!), volunteering, or even participating in a good old-fashioned game of their favorite team activity (more on this later). Just remember, teamwork makes the dream work.

"It is the long history of humankind (and animal kind, too) that those who learned to collaborate and improvise most effectively have prevailed."

~ Charles Darwin

Collaboration isn't just limited to group activities outside of the home. You can also foster collaboration within the family unit. For instance, involve your teen in family decisions, like what to have for dinner or which movie to watch on family night (good luck!).

Let's be real, as parents, we can also benefit from some team-building exercises. We could start a family game night or maybe even try to tackle a home improvement project together. Who knows, we may even learn a thing or two from our teens! And this way, they can understand the practical application, as well as the importance of collaboration.

By emphasizing collaboration, we are not only helping our teens develop the skills they need to succeed but also preparing them for future leadership roles. After all, we could all use a little help from our teammates every now and then.

Collaboration is no ordinary ingredient in the recipe for success. It's the spice that propels our teenagers beyond their limits, allowing them to achieve feats they could never accomplish alone and build strong relationships with those around them.

But why is collaboration so important in personal growth and leadership development? Allow me to elaborate. When teenagers collaborate, they have to put into practice and learn the art of effective communication, active listening, and empathy. They develop the skills to navigate wide-ranging opinions and find common ground, fostering an inclusive and harmonious environment where everyone's voices are heard.

Collaboration also breeds innovation and creativity. When minds come together, ideas collide, and sparks ignite. By encouraging our kids to collaborate, we might just help them unlock a treasure trove of innovative solutions and ground-breaking initiatives. Through collaboration, they learn to think outside the box, challenge conventional wisdom, and potentially create something that surpasses their wildest dreams.

The beauty of collaboration goes beyond just the end result, it is about the things we learn on the journey because when teenagers collaborate, they build strong relationships based on trust, respect, and shared goals. They learn the art of compromise, conflict resolution, and teamwork.

The Power Of "We" In Leadership

First and foremost, collaboration creates a sense of shared ownership and engagement. Leaders who promote collaboration cultivate a culture where everyone's vantage points and contributions are highly valued. This inclusive approach boosts motivation and strengthens commitment toward shared goals. By actively involving team members in decision-making processes, leaders tap into their collective wisdom and expertise, ultimately leading to better outcomes, which improves the way teams work together and solve problems.

"Cooperation is the thorough conviction that nobody can get there unless everybody gets there."

~ Virginia Burden

Collaboration fuels creativity and innovation because when individuals with eclectic backgrounds and skill sets collaborate, they bring unique insights and ideas to the table. Teams can leverage this diversity to generate innovative solutions for complex problems, through collaborative efforts. The fusion of different viewpoints often ignites creativity, stimulates unconventional thinking, and opens doors to ground breaking discoveries.

By prioritizing collaboration, leaders create an environment of open communication and mutual respect. Team members feel valued, heard, and understood, which strengthens their bond and cultivates a sense of camaraderie. Trust flourishes as individuals rely on each other's expertise, share responsibilities, and offer support.

Furthermore, collaboration facilitates learning and professional growth. By collaborating with others, individuals gain access to a wealth of knowledge and experiences beyond their own. They have the opportunity to learn from their peers, acquire new skills, and broaden their horizons. Leaders who foster collaboration provide team members with valuable opportunities for development, fostering a culture of continuous learning.

In today's interconnected and complex world, no single leader possesses all the answers or skills required to tackle multifaceted challenges. By fostering collaboration, leaders unlock the power of synergy, resulting in enhanced problem-solving abilities, greater adaptability, and improved organizational performance.

Practical Steps For Encouraging Collaboration

If you want your teenagers to grow up and become successful leaders, you gotta teach 'em how to collaborate. I mean, it's not just about working well with others. Collaboration can help them build strong relationships, learn how to communicate effectively, and develop important social skills. And let's face it, they're gonna need all of those things to survive in this mad world.

How do you inspire collaboration among teens? Simple. You provide them with opportunities to work with others, like activity days, group projects, team sports, or even just hanging out with their friends and giving them a challenge to solve. If they argue or fight, use it as a teachable moment to help them learn how to resolve conflicts and share responsibilities.

By equipping our teens with all these valuable skills, we provide them with the necessary tools to become transformative leaders who can make a significant impact on the world. And isn't that what we want for our kids? Let's take a look at some actionable steps to prompt our teens to collaborate:

1. Creating a cooperative environment: If you want to raise a collaboration-savvy teenager, highlight the power of teamwork and cooperation in achieving shared goals. It's all about setting the stage and making sure they know the ground rules for collaborative behavior, like being an active participant, giving mad respect to other people's ideas, and being open to the art of compromise. By putting these guidelines in place, we create a safe and welcoming space where everyone feels like a valued player on the team. Here are a couple of fun and practical activities, that I've learned over the years raising Noah.

Boo The Dragon:

This is good for larger groups that can compete in smaller teams. The aim of this game is for the teams to arrange themselves according to their height, all while being blindfolded, and as fast as possible. It necessitates cooperation and a touch of creativity.

Break the group into even teams, while one teen is the dragon (the judge). The teams can discuss the approach once the dragon says "Go". The first team who thinks they're in the correct order, shouts "Boo" to scare the dragon. The dragon judges if they're in proper order, and the first team to line up correctly wins. It may seem like a silly game, but it really gets teens thinking differently and communicating.

If that's not your thing, or you want a different kind of mental challenge for a smaller group, try "The Egg Drop". This challenge basically involves two teams with equal resources and standing on a chair to drop an egg – the aim of the game (particularly if playing at your house!) is to not have your egg crack and break. You can give each team newspaper (or tissues), straws, rubber bands, tape, and small cardboard boxes or cardboard tubes. This is just a suggestion. One of the great things about this activity is that you can use whatever materials you want. The only limit is its ability to keep an egg from breaking. This one gets them communicating and trying to problem-solve creatively.

2. Developing effective communication skills: In Chapter 2, we looked at Effective Communication Skills. Killer collaboration skills require effective communication skills, so we're refreshing a little here. First up, we gotta school them in the art of active listening. This is all about tuning in, understanding and resisting the temptation to butt in with their assumptions (because nobody likes a know-it-all, right?). Before they take on any teamwork tasks, we can give them a crash course in communication finesse, both in what they say and how they say it. Clear and concise expression wins hands down here, combined with the power of constructive feedback and open dialogue. When they embrace these gems, they'll become masters of healthy discussions, problem-solving, and making decisions together with their peers as a united front.

3. Promoting diversity and inclusion: Encouraging your teenager to embrace multifarious perspectives and value differences is another imperative along the path to fostering collaboration. We can challenge them to step outside their comfort zones and engage with people from different backgrounds, cultures, and experiences. By creating opportunities for cross-cultural and interdisciplinary collaboration, such as group projects or joint activities, we provide platforms for teenagers to learn from one another and appreciate the strength that comes from diversity. This cultivates an environment where collaboration thrives through the richness of varied ideas and interpretations.

4. Facilitating group projects and team-building activities: One surefire way to get your teenager flexing their teamwork muscles is by dishing out some collaborative tasks. Yep, handing them a challenge that requires their superpowers of coordination, communication, and leveraging strengths with others so that they'll learn the art of creating a well-oiled machine, delegating tasks and working together towards that sweet, sweet taste of success. So, rouse them to dive into group projects at school or join extracurricular activities that require collaboration. Not only will they learn how to work like a dynamic duo (or trio or more), but they'll also get a chance to sharpen their leadership skills and forge awesome relationships with their peers. We also can't overlook the significance of the power of team-building activities. Whether it's tackling outdoor challenges or cracking their brains with problem-solving games, these activities are like bonding glue. They'll build trust, cooperation, and those ever-so-important problem-solving skills. Before you know it, your teenager and their co-collaborators will be armed with camaraderie and ready to conquer any collaboration mission that comes their way!

5. Team sports or clubs: Spur your teen to join a team sport or club. This not only promotes physical fitness and personal development but also provides valuable opportunities for collaboration. Being part of a team sport or club helps

teenagers learn how to work together towards a shared goal, whether scoring a goal, creating a performance, or organizing an event. They develop essential teamwork skills, such as effective communication, cooperation, and coordination. Moreover, being part of a team or club fosters a sense of belonging and camaraderie, allowing teenagers to experience the power of collective effort and the satisfaction of achieving success together.

By implementing these practical steps, we create an environment that fosters collaboration, such as valuing teamwork, developing effective communication skills, promoting diversity and inclusion, and facilitating group projects and team-building activities, to equip our teens with the necessary tools to collaborate successfully. Collaboration becomes not only a means to achieve common goals but also a mentality and approach that can lead to innovative solutions, increased productivity, and a sense of collective achievement.

Noah's Story About Collaboration / Teamwork

At the age of 10, Noah discovered the power of collaboration and harnessed it through an unexpected avenue: building a Discord server. Eager to create a thriving online community for gamers, Noah realized he couldn't tackle all the tasks alone. Instead, he embraced his entrepreneurial spirit and turned to Fiverr, a freelancing platform, to seek assistance for each challenge he faced. With determination and a budget of $5 per task, Noah began to assemble a team of experts.

As Noah encountered obstacles beyond his skillset, he hired programmers, designers, and other professionals to complete each specific task. With each successful collaboration, Noah not only learned how to effectively manage his team but also witnessed the remarkable outcomes that synergy could achieve. By promoting open communication and fostering a sense of unity among his team members, Noah ensured everyone's strengths were maximized, leading to efficient and productive progress.

Remarkably, Noah's strategic approach and dedication to collaboration allowed him to accomplish his ambitious goals within a month, all while staying within his modest budget of $35. Through this experience, Noah not only honed his technical skills but also developed valuable leadership qualities. This early exposure to teamwork and effective project management would become the foundation for his future endeavors, showcasing the immense power of collaboration and its potential to achieve remarkable outcomes even at a young age.

Final Thoughts On Encouraging Collaboration In Your Teenager

Collaboration isn't just some fancy term tossed around in boring business meetings or tedious school projects. By reinforcing the significance of collaboration, we're showing them that authentic leadership isn't about flying solo or hogging the spotlight. It's about coming together, harnessing the power of broad-ranging approaches, and achieving greatness as a team.

When we promote collaboration, we're not just promoting teamwork for the sake of getting things done. No, no, no. We're unleashing a whole world of innovation, creativity, and collective success. It's like mixing a bunch of vibrant colors on a canvas and creating a masterpiece that nobody could have achieved alone. Collaboration breeds ideas, sparks inspiration, and pushes boundaries. It's where the magic happens that makes our teams go from "meh" to "epic." When we work together, we can achieve anything. It's all about creating a culture of openness, respect, and trust, which, incidentally, is precisely what you need with your teen.

We need to teach our teens (and teams) to listen like never before because when we listen, we can understand each other's mindsets and work towards a common goal. We also need to motivate our teens to be respectful, even when they disagree. Like the age-old adage, "Treat others the way you want to be treated." When we show respect, we can create a safe and supportive environment for everyone to share their ideas.

Let's inspire our teenagers to embrace collaboration as a valuable skill for their personal and professional growth. Let them see the power of synergy, where the sum is greater than its parts. Empower them to step outside their comfort zones, seek out diverse perspectives, and value the unique contributions on offer. In doing so, we're preparing them not only for success but also for a fulfilling and connected life.

Chapter 13: Yo, I need some help here: Unlocking the Power of Delegation

Delegation, baby! It's the thing that takes a great idea and makes it scalable! And yeah, even teenagers can rock at it. We're going to talk about raising teenagers who know how to delegate like pros. Delegation isn't just about passing off tasks like a hot potato (although that's definitely a perk). Delegation is a skill that can transform teens and young leaders, helping them grow, build trust, and make a real impact.

"If you want to do a few small things right, do them yourself. If you want to do great things and make a big impact, learn to delegate."

~ John C. Maxwell

So, why is delegation so damn important? Well, teenagers have a million things on their plates - school, sports, clubs, you name it, and they need to learn how to get stuff done without burning out. That's where delegation swoops in. It lets them tap into the strengths and talents of their friends, peers, teams, and clubs, multiplying their productivity and saving their sanity.

Picture a teenage leader with a mountain of tasks piled high like a Jenga tower on the brink of collapse. By entrusting tasks to capable team members, leaders can focus their precious time and energy on higher-level responsibilities. It's like having a personal army of minions (minus the evil villain vibes) to handle the nitty-gritty while leaders tackle the strategic big picture. Productivity soars, efficiency reigns, and everyone cheers—well, maybe not everyone, but you get the idea.

Delegation isn't just about checking boxes on a to-do list. As our kids grow up, they are exposed to new challenges and new opportunities. Delegation is a chance for teenagers to develop their communication skills, stimulate teamwork, and solve problems. By passing the baton to their teammates, they're giving them room to shine, grow, and take ownership of their work. It's like building a dream team.

Throughout this chapter, we'll lay out some practical steps for our teens and future leaders to become delegation gurus. We'll talk about assessing tasks, empowering the team, and being the supportive parental figure they need. Oh, and we'll cover the secret of delegation – trust. Because without trust, well, it's like trying to swim without water. Let's show them how to change the game and make things happen. It's delegation time, baby!

Why Effective Delegation Is Important In Leadership

First and foremost, delegating allows leaders to focus their time and energy on what truly matters. By delegating tasks to their team, they free up precious mental bandwidth and create space for strategic thinking, decision-making, and big-picture visioning. That allows them to step into the leadership zone, where they can make a real impact.

Delegation isn't just a one-way street. Effective delegation is a recipe for building trust and fostering a positive team culture. When leaders trust their team members with important responsibilities, it sends a powerful message - "I believe in you, and I value your contribution." It creates a sense of ownership and empowerment, fueling motivation and engagement. And when the team feels trusted and appreciated, they step up, bring their best to the table, and unleash their full potential.

Delegation fosters open communication, creating an environment where team members can share ideas, insights, and the occasional cat video. It's about building trust and unity, like a team huddling together for a victory chant (minus the sweat and awkward high fives). Together, they conquer mountains, slay dragons, and—oh wait, sorry, got carried away there. But you get the point.

Effective delegation is not just about the immediate benefits but also the long-term impact it has on leadership development. It's a skill that teenagers can carry with them throughout their lives in any endeavor they pursue. Whether they become entrepreneurs, managers, or community leaders, the ability to delegate effectively will set them apart and propel them toward success.

Leadership isn't a one-and-done gig, either. It's also about passing the baton. Effective delegation plays a central role in grooming the next leaders that follow, and this is something your teen can find opportunities to do in sports teams, clubs, and community groups. So, with that in mind, let's look at some effective steps for developing delegation skills in your teenager.

Practical Steps To Help Your Teenager To Become A Master Of Effective Delegation

Helping your teenager become a master of effective delegation can equip them with valuable skills in time management, leadership, and beyond. Here are some practical steps you can take to support them in this process:

1. Assessing tasks and responsibilities: Before teenagers jump into the wild world of delegation, they need to put on their detective hats and do some serious task evaluation. Think of it as a leadership version of "CSI: Delegation Edition." They must examine each task and responsibility, separating the delegation-worthy gems from the ones better left to the experts. They also need to gauge the level of responsibility required for each job. Some tasks may be like free-range

chickens, needing just a little nudge in the right direction. Others, however, might be like mischievous puppies, requiring constant attention and guidance. It's all about finding that sweet spot of oversight.

2. Lead by example: One powerful way to showcase the power of delegation to your teenager is by embodying it yourself. Take the initiative to delegate tasks within the family, and make a conscious effort to explain your thought process behind each delegation. For instance, you can assign household chores, such as cleaning or organizing, to different family members based on their strengths and interests. As you delegate, openly discuss why you chose a specific task for each person, emphasizing how their skills align with the task at hand. By doing so, you not only set a positive example but also provide your teenager with valuable insight into the reasoning behind delegation and how it can lead to shared responsibilities and a more harmonious household.

3. Explain the benefits: Sit down with your teenager for an open and (hopefully) enlightening conversation about the advantages of delegation. Paint a vivid picture of how it can be a time-saver and rescue precious minutes from the clutches of mundane tasks. Discuss how delegation boosts efficiency, curbs micromanaging, and acts as a turbocharger for productivity by leveraging the skills and abilities of others. Highlight how it liberates others to learn new skills as it allows them to shift their focus to more

important or enjoyable tasks that align with their passions and personal growth.

4. Assess and select suitable individuals: Emphasize how this strategic matching of tasks to people's strengths leads to better outcomes, whether it's achieving goals more efficiently or delivering exceptional results. Highlight the ripple effect that delegation can have on personal growth, as both the delegate and the delegator learn from each other, broaden their skill sets, and gain new perspectives. Our teens can learn to become masters of task matchmaking, skillfully assigning responsibilities to the individuals who possess the ideal combination of expertise and enthusiasm, and unleash the full potential of their team, or group.

5. Start small: Begin with small, manageable tasks that your teenager feels comfortable delegating. This helps build confidence and demonstrates the positive results that come from sharing the workload. Choose tasks that are manageable and within their comfort zone, ensuring they don't feel overwhelmed or anxious about the process. By beginning small, you create an environment where they can build confidence in their delegation abilities, one task at a time. This gradual approach sets the stage for your teenager to develop the skills and mindset necessary for effective delegation on a larger scale in the future. Watch their confidence and trust in the power of

shared responsibilities grow with each accomplished task.

6. Provide guidance: Become a guide and mentor to your teenager as you teach them the art of effectively communicating tasks to be delegated, focusing on clear instructions and expectations. Emphasize the importance of expressing their needs and desired outcomes with clarity, as if they were crafting a message in a bottle destined for success. Teach them to anticipate potential challenges and address them proactively by offering guidance, insights, or access to relevant tools or information. By instilling these communication skills, you empower your teenager to create a supportive and efficient environment for delegation, where everyone involved understands the expectations and has the necessary resources to succeed.

7. Offer feedback and support: As your teenager ventures into the realm of delegation, be their unwavering support system, providing feedback and guidance along the way. Embolden them to seek feedback from the individuals to whom they delegate tasks, like an inquisitive explorer seeking insights from fellow adventurers. This feedback becomes a valuable compass, guiding them towards improvement and refinement in their delegation skills. Be there to offer your own guidance and insights, drawing from your own experiences.

Final Thoughts On Effective Delegation In Raising Leaders

We've traversed this chapter like a majestic river flowing through the meandering valleys of leadership. Let's take a moment to recap the key concepts and steps we've covered on this delegation journey.

We started by assessing tasks and responsibilities, sorting through the chaos like a teenager on a decluttering spree, or maybe that should be a cluttering spree, seems more apt! We helped our teens identify what COULD be delegated, leaving them with a lighter load to carry, and then, like talent scouts, they handpicked suitable individuals for each task, matching skills and interests. Then they stepped it up a notch to communicate expectations clearly, making sure everyone was on the same page—no cryptic hieroglyphics allowed.

Next, we empowered our teens to trust their team members, giving them the space to shine and trusting them with the power to make decisions. The glue that holds it all together? Setting deadlines and milestones, not with a whip, but with a gentle, yet direct nudge, and a sprinkle of encouragement. Our teens can learn to create a feedback loop, like a communication highway, allowing them to monitor progress and guide their peers and team members toward greatness.

Chapter 14: Foster Innovation

Welcome to our penultimate chapter, numero 14. Innovation is all about thinking outside the box, pushing boundaries, and coming up with fresh ideas that make the world go, "Holy moly, that's awesome!" And guess what? Teenagers have a unique advantage when it comes to innovation. Their minds are think tanks of creativity, churning out ideas faster than you can say, "Supercalifragilisticexpialidocious!?"

Why is innovation important in the world of leadership? Well, imagine you're at a party, and there are two types of people there. You've got your run-of-the-mill partygoers who stick to the same old dance moves and conversation topics. And then, you've got the innovators, the ones who break out the robot dance moves, and come up with mind-blowing party tricks. Who do you think everyone's going to remember? Exactly! The innovators steal the show and leave everyone wanting more.

The same principle applies to leadership. Leaders who can guide themselves and their teams into and through innovation, stand out from the crowd. It's what separates the leaders who make waves from the ones who just bob along with the current. Innovative leaders drive progress and success in their fields. They're the ones who disrupt industries, create ground breaking solutions, and leave their competitors scratching their heads in awe.

"Creativity is thinking up new things. Innovation is doing new things."

~ Theodore Levitt

Innovation isn't just for the tech wizards or the Steve Jobs of the world. It's for each and every kid who wants to make a difference, leave a mark, and have a damn good time while doing it.

In this chapter, we'll undertake an in-depth exploration into the practical steps, the whys, and the hows of fostering innovation in our teenagers to help them adapt to change and keep moving forward, both in life and in their endeavors. We'll explore the power of thinking differently, embracing creativity, making a positive impact, and more.

Igniting The Spark: Unleashing The Power Of Innovation In Leadership

Innovation is about driving progress and staying ahead of the curve. In a world that's constantly evolving, leaders who embrace innovation can adapt to changing circumstances and seize new opportunities with agility and finesse. They're unafraid to challenge the status quo and push the boundaries of what's possible. By fostering a culture of innovation, leaders ensure that their teams and organizations remain relevant, competitive, and at the forefront of progress.

What happens when leaders prioritize and cultivate a culture of innovation and creativity? They create an enthusiastic team bursting with creative energy and bold ideas. They understand that innovation thrives in an atmosphere of psychological safety, where team members feel empowered to take risks and learn from failures. Solving complex problems and making a positive impact is key. By nurturing a culture of innovation, leaders unleash the collective brilliance of their team and create a breeding ground for breakthrough ideas.

The world is full of complicated issues just waiting to be solved. From environmental challenges to social inequality, innovative leaders have the power to tackle these issues head-on and find creative solutions.

What's more, smart leaders can take a difficult task and apply a value to it to help motivate their team. For example, imagine you're working on a complex problem or project. As a team, you know working on this problem will involve countless sleepless nights and a hell of a lot of constant work and effort. You're wondering if it's really worth it? Now, imagine your leader telling you it's worth an extra $8 million to find the right system to manage the problem or, even better, solve it. Seems way more worth investigating now, right?

Teenagers are not just the leaders of tomorrow; they are the leaders in the making today. By empowering them to think innovatively, we can equip teenagers with the skills, mindset, and confidence they need to become effective leaders in their chosen fields. We can instill in them the belief that they have the power to make a difference, challenge the status quo, and drive positive change as a generation of change-makers who will shape the future and leave an indelible mark on the world.

Spark The Genius: Unleash Innovation In Your Teen With Practical Steps

Let's get down to business and talk about how we can create an environment that facilitates creativity and curiosity. We're going to turn your family space into an innovation playground where experimentation and risk-taking are not only welcomed but celebrated with high-fives, fist bumps, and the odd grilled cheese waffle...mmm...grilled cheese. Did you know that it was an American with Dutch heritage (obviously) who patented the first modern waffle iron back in 1869? Cornelius Swartwout created a stove-top version of the waffle iron that was easy to turn and less likely to burn the hand of the cook. And it also birthed another game-changing idea that made a lasting impact on contemporary culture: the athletic shoe. In 1972, Bill Bowerman, a track coach from the University of Oregon, sought a patent for a groundbreaking sports footwear concept. He introduced shaped rubber studs on the sole to enhance traction, ingeniously using his wife's waffle iron to create a distinctive grip pattern. With that, Bowerman, who would go on to establish Nike, was off and running. Now, that's innovation! Sorry, I'm hungry, and I digress. Let's crack on…

Break the rules, baby! Innovation thrives when rules are meant to be bent, twisted, and occasionally tossed out the window altogether. Elicit your teenager to think outside the box, challenge the status quo, and dare to do things differently. Let them know that it's okay to color outside the lines and that mistakes are just stepping stones on the path to brilliance.

Embrace the power of continuous learning: Curiosity is like a muscle, and it needs to be flexed regularly. Create a culture where learning is not just a chore but an exciting adventure. Inspire your teenager to devour books on topics they love, explore new ideas, and dive headfirst into subjects that ignite their curiosity. Let them know that knowledge is powerful and that the more they learn, the more they can innovate.

Provide resources for exploration: Innovation needs fuel, and that fuel comes in the form of resources. Equip your teenager with the tools they need to unleash their creativity. Whether it's apps, books, online courses, or access to experts in their field of interest, give them the keys to the kingdom of knowledge.

Treat failure with the same enthusiasm as success:

Alfred Nobel, the Swedish chemist, engineer, inventor, businessman, and philanthropist, who held 355 patents in his lifetime, made several important scientific contributions and left his fortune to establish the Nobel Prize once said, "If I have 1,000 ideas and only one turns out to be good, I am satisfied." Innovation and failure go hand in hand. Let your teenager know that it's okay to stumble and fall on their path and bolster them to take risks. Throw a failure party if you have to, complete with balloons and a piñata filled with lessons learned. Failure is not the end; it's just a detour on the road to innovation.

Provide Opportunities For Problem-Solving And Critical Thinking

When we encourage teenagers to dive into problem-solving activities, we're giving them a chance to sharpen their practical skills. They learn to dissect complex situations, think critically, and emerge with solutions that make the world go, "Wow, that's impressive!" It's not just about being book-smart.

Engaging in activities that require them to analyze situations, think critically, and devise effective solutions equips them with practical skills applicable to various aspects of their lives. Additionally, these experiences foster adaptability, enabling teenagers to navigate challenges and changes with confidence.

Encouraging independent problem-solving builds their self-reliance, decision-making abilities, and sense of ownership. So, let's look at how to do this:

Bring on the brain teasers! Give your teenager puzzles (personally, I like the Sudoku Puzzle books or anxiety relief word searches for teens and adults by "Mental Spark" on

Amazon), riddles, and mind-bending challenges that make their neurons tango. Whether it's a Rubik's Cube, a complex mathematical problem, or a perplexing brainteaser, these challenges will stretch their cognitive muscles and train their brains to think outside the box. Think of it as mental gymnastics with a touch of genius.

Real-world problems, meet teenage superheroes: Give your teenager a chance to solve real-world problems that matter. Present them with challenges that align with their interests and passions, whether it's tackling environmental issues, addressing social inequalities, or inventing the next revolutionary gadget. Let them unleash their innovative ideas and watch them transform into problem-solving creativity machines.

Rouse them to think like Sherlock Holmes: Critical thinking is all about examining the evidence, connecting the dots, and arriving at logical conclusions. Teach your teenager the art of deduction (my dear Watson!). Show them how to gather information, analyze different perspectives, and evaluate the pros and cons of potential solutions. Channel their inner detective and let them navigate the labyrinth of problem-solving with finesse.

Fail forward: Innovation and problem-solving are not always smooth sailing. Sometimes you hit dead ends, encounter setbacks, or end up with solutions that need a little tweaking. Embrace the beauty of trial and error, and enliven your teenager to see setbacks as stepping stones, even the ones that don't quite go according to plan. Remember, the greatest inventors and problem solvers were not deterred by failure but FUELED BY IT!

Foster a culture of curiosity and exploration: Travel, go camping, or go to a museum. Wonder out loud, for example, I wonder why the sky and sea are both blue? Prompt thinking, when your kid asks you a question, ask them their thoughts before answering. It was Albert Einstein who, in Life magazine, wrote that "The important thing is not to stop questioning; curiosity has its own reason for existing. One cannot help but be in awe when contemplating the mysteries of eternity, of life, of the marvelous structure of reality. It is enough if one tries merely to comprehend a little of the mystery every day. The important thing is not to stop questioning; never lose a holy curiosity."

Curiosity is the fuel that powers problem-solving and critical thinking. Between you and I, it is my personal belief that it gets a bit of a bad rap, and did most certainly NOT kill the cat. Endorse asking questions, seeking answers, and exploring different perspectives to instill in them that the world is their intellectual playground, and their questions are the keys that unlock the doors of innovation. Even if it did kill the cat, it surely birthed some incredible inventions in the process.

Advocate For Collaboration And Diverse Perspectives

In the grand tapestry of our interconnected world, my friend, advocating for collaboration and diverse perspectives among our teenagers is nothing short of essential. By crafting environments that foster collaboration, we gift them a gateway to interact with individuals from diverse backgrounds, cultures, and experiences. And let me tell you, it's a recipe for enhanced creativity that'll make their mind explode with possibilities! How, do I hear you cry? Well, honestly, I can't actually hear anything right now, except incessant ringing in my ears… terrible incident involving my proximity to fireworks last night, but anyway, here are some ideas on how:

Stir up collaboration and idea-sharing: Innovation is a team sport. Foster an environment where your teenager can collaborate in groups, clubs, and teams, wherever the opportunity arises, for them to bounce ideas off others and build upon one another's brilliance. Create spaces for brainstorming sessions, group projects, and lively discussions. Remember, the more minds you bring together, the more innovative the ideas that will emerge.

Embrace the beauty of diversity: It's time to celebrate the vibrant tapestry of perspectives and ideas. Incite your teen to seek out diverse voices and opinions. Whether it's through eclectic reading materials, engaging with people from different backgrounds, or attending multicultural events, expose them to a world of diverse perspectives. Remind them that innovation thrives when it is nurtured by a rich blend of ideas from various cultures, backgrounds, and experiences.

Break down the barriers: Create an inclusive and welcoming environment where every voice is valued and heard. A culture that facilitates active listening, empathy, and respect for differing viewpoints. Teach your teenager the art of constructive feedback and open-mindedness. By creating a safe space for expression, you'll unleash the full potential of their collaborative powers.

Think beyond boundaries: Support interdisciplinary collaboration that transcends traditional silos. Break down the walls between different subjects and disciplines, and let your teenager explore the intersection of pluralistic fields. When science meets art, when technology meets social activism, and when creativity merges with analytical thinking, that's where true innovation thrives. Inspire your teen to think beyond boundaries and embrace the exciting possibilities that arise from interdisciplinary collaboration.

Fuel their entrepreneurial fire: Identify and provide the necessary resources and support for their entrepreneurial ventures. Help them access relevant information, books, online courses, and workshops that can sharpen their business acumen. Embolden them to explore different business models, marketing strategies, and financial management techniques. Remember, knowledge is power, and a well-informed teenage entrepreneur is a force to be reckoned with.

Guide them through the entrepreneurial journey: Starting a business can be like riding a roller coaster blindfolded! Be there to provide guidance and support as your teenage entrepreneurs navigate the ups and downs of their ventures. Help them develop business plans, set goals, and establish strategies for growth. Fortify them to embrace failure as a learning opportunity and to adapt and pivot when needed. Remember, even the most successful entrepreneurs have faced setbacks and obstacles along their journeys.

Stimulating Creativity Through Art, Technology, And Design

Ah, the vast and wondrous realm of creativity! Within it lies a trifecta that can ignite the fire within our teenagers: art, technology, and design. Through the avenue of artistic expression, we grant them the freedom to unleash their innermost thoughts and emotions, allowing their imagination to soar unfettered. Simultaneously, the marvels of technology unveil a vast playground where they can explore coding, programming, graphic design, and digital media, unlocking a world of endless possibilities. And when they don the lens of design, they become architects of their reality, transforming intangible ideas into tangible, meaningful creations. The stimulation of creativity through art, technology, and design not only offers a gateway to unlimited potential but also empowers our teenagers to leave an indelible mark on the tapestry of innovation and beauty that surrounds us.

Embrace the artistry: Introduce your teenager to various forms of artistic expression, from painting and drawing to music and dance. Inspire them to explore different art mediums and techniques, allowing their imagination to run wild. Art provides a powerful outlet for creativity, allowing teenagers to express their thoughts, emotions, and unique perspectives. Who knows, your teenager might become the next Picasso or Beyoncé!

Embrace technology: In today's digital age, technology plays a pivotal role in innovation and problem-solving. Spur your teenager on to explore technology as a tool for creativity and innovation. From coding and programming to graphic design and app development, technology opens up a world of possibilities for them to bring their ideas to life. They might even create the next ground breaking app that solves everyday problems or revolutionizes an industry. The sky's the limit!

Design the future: Design thinking is all about problem-solving and creating user-centered solutions. Rouse your teenager to embrace design as a pathway to innovation. Introduce them to design thinking principles, where they can empathize with users, define problems, ideate solutions, prototype, and iterate. Design can be applied to various fields, from product design to user experience (UX) design, and even designing social initiatives.

Provide opportunities for exploration: Create an environment where teenagers can freely explore their artistic, technological, and design interests. Organize workshops, field trips, or, if available, guest speaker sessions to expose them to professionals in these fields. Encourage them to attend art exhibits, technology conferences, or design competitions. By immersing themselves in these experiences, they can gain inspiration, expand their horizons, and discover their unique creative talents.

Embrace the fusion of art, technology, and design: Support your teenager to embrace the intersection of art, technology, and design. Show them examples of how these fields converge to create innovative and impactful projects. From interactive installations to virtual reality experiences, the fusion of art, technology, and design can push boundaries and revolutionize industries. Help your teen to think beyond the traditional silos and explore how they can integrate these disciplines into their own creative endeavors.

Final Thoughts On Fostering Innovation

As we wrap up this chapter on encouraging innovation in our teens, let's take a moment to reflect on the transformative power of embracing innovation.

First and foremost, remember that innovation is not reserved for the elite few or the geniuses among us. It's a spark that resides in each and every one of us, waiting to be ignited. So, let's be fearless in our pursuit of new ideas and solutions. Let's not be afraid to challenge the norms, question the status quo, and push the boundaries of what's possible. Innovation thrives when we dare to step outside our comfort zones and explore uncharted territories.

Teenagers have a unique advantage when it comes to innovation. Their fresh perspective, unencumbered by years of conformity, allows them to see possibilities where others see obstacles. They have the audacity to dream big, to think differently, and to reimagine the world around them. It's our duty to nurture and channel this untapped potential by providing them with the tools and guidance to think creatively.

Innovation is not a one-time event; it's a lifelong pursuit. It requires continuous learning, adaptation, and evolution. We must foster a culture that values and rewards innovation. We must create spaces where ideas can flourish, where experimentation is encouraged, and where failures are seen as steps on the path to success.

Chapter 15: Sharing Knowledge

(Teaching and Training Others)

Remember when you first started driving a car? It's been so long that you probably forgot. Well, let me jog your memory. Sweaty palms. Racing heart. The first car you ever had the chance to drive was probably your parents' or a friend's, in an empty parking lot. They were probably there on the passenger side, giving you tips and guidance while simultaneously holding on for dear life. It may have taken a few hours or maybe a few days, but with their patient training, you eventually got there. Now look at you, cursing at incompetent drivers on the road, proud of your driving skills... or, at least so competent that the majority of them have become subconscious!

Empowering others through teaching and training is a game-changer, my friend. It's like creating a ripple effect of growth and development that reaches far beyond our immediate circles. Think about it: Remember when your parent or friend taught you how to drive? That's exactly what they did, they empowered you. Gave you the confidence or capability to do well in something you had no knowledge about before. And here's the beautiful part: They also granted you the opportunity to pay it forward, to pass on that knowledge and empower others, perhaps even your own teenager.

"The greatest gift you can give someone is the power to be successful. Giving opens the way for receiving."

~ Jon Bon Jovi

Teaching and training nurture a growth mindset in teenagers. It teaches them that knowledge is not fixed or limited but rather something that can be deepened through the continuous sharing of it. Furthermore, sharing knowledge builds confidence and self-esteem in teenagers. When they witness the impact of their teachings and the positive reception of their efforts, they develop a sense of accomplishment and belief in their own abilities. They realize that their voice matters and that they have valuable insights to offer to others.

"The best way to learn is to teach."

~ Frank Oppenheimer

In this chapter, we will explore practical techniques and strategies for effective teaching and training. We will delve into the importance of understanding individual learning styles, developing communication, and honing presentation skills. We will also discuss the significance of mentoring relationships, peer-to-peer learning, and community involvement in creating meaningful opportunities for teenagers to share their knowledge and make a positive impact on society at large.

"Share your knowledge. It is a way to achieve immortality." - Dalai Lama

Why Sharing Knowledge Is Important In Leadership

Leaders who grasp the significance of sharing their wisdom and experiences unlock a world of potential. They create an environment that becomes fertile soil for personal and professional growth. By generously imparting their expertise, skills, and experiences, leaders become catalysts for the advancement of their team members. They understand that when knowledge flows freely, it multiplies, elevating everyone involved. It's a beautiful dance of knowledge as leaders become both teachers and students, and team members become both learners and contributors.

When leaders are transparent and accessible, they create an atmosphere of trust where team members feel comfortable seeking guidance, asking questions, and sharing ideas. By actively engaging in knowledge sharing, leaders lay the foundation for strong, cohesive teams where everyone feels valued and contributes to collective success.

Sharing knowledge also empowers and motivates others. When leaders share their expertise, they equip team members with the tools and resources needed to excel in their roles. This empowerment fuels motivation, as individuals feel valued, supported, and confident in their abilities. Remember the saying "Competence breeds Confidence"? It also cultivates a sense of autonomy, enabling team members to make informed decisions and contribute meaningfully to the team's objectives without needing direct managerial oversight. By empowering others, leaders foster a sense of ownership and accountability, which leads to higher levels of engagement and performance.

Furthermore, sharing knowledge strengthens relationships and communication within a team. I mean, who doesn't wanna get leveled up? Leaders establish a bond built on trust and understanding by being open and transparent in what they know. The strengthened relationships facilitate collaboration and create a positive work environment where everyone feels not just heard and valued, but enhanced.

"Knowledge is power. Information is liberating. Education is the premise of progress, in every society, in every family." - Kofi Annan

Sharing knowledge isn't just about personal and team growth; it's also a strategic move for the future. They understand that a well-prepared successor means a future leader who can step into their role with confidence and competence. This deliberate knowledge transfer bridges any potential gaps and maintains the momentum of progress within a professional organization, sports team, or even family.

Practical Approaches For Inspiring Your Teen To Share What They Know

Nurturing Intellectual Curiosity: Sharing knowledge cultivates and nourishes the inherent curiosity that resides within all of us, our transitional young adults included. It sparks a desire to seek understanding, question the world around them, and explore new realms of knowledge. By providing them with access to information, insights, and experiences, we fuel their intellectual growth and ignite a passion for lifelong learning. When we have a genuine love for something, we almost can't help but share it.

As we engage teenagers in the act of sharing knowledge, we energize them to ask questions, challenge assumptions, and think critically. We empower them to be active participants in their own learning journey, fostering a sense of ownership and agency over their education.

Fostering Confidence and Self-Esteem: When teenagers take on the role of teachers and trainers, they experience a profound boost in their confidence and self-esteem. As they share their knowledge and expertise, they witness the impact their words and actions have on others. This validation reinforces their belief in their own abilities and strengthens their sense of self-worth.

Through teaching and training, teenagers develop communication and presentation skills, enabling them to articulate their thoughts and ideas with clarity and conviction. They learn to organize their knowledge, structure their presentations, and engage their audience. As they witness the positive reception of their teachings, their confidence soars, and they gain a newfound belief in their capacity to make a difference.

Cultivating Leadership Skills: Within this domain, sharing knowledge holds a vital position. Through teaching and training, teenagers refine their abilities as leaders, encompassing crucial traits like effective communication, empathy, and the power to inspire and influence others for the better. In this process, they acquire the skill to tailor their teaching methods to suit varied audiences, adapting their approach to cater to the distinct requirements of individuals and groups. By elucidating and simplifying concepts for others, they deepen their own understanding of the subject matter. In addition, they learn to modify their teaching style to accommodate broad-ranging learning preferences, fostering an environment that promotes inclusivity and support.

Deepening Understanding and Mastery: When teenagers teach and train others, they deepen their own understanding and mastery of the subject matter. As they explain concepts, answer questions, and provide guidance, they must engage with the material on a deeper level. This process of articulating and teaching reinforces their own knowledge and allows them to identify any gaps in their understanding.

Through the act of teaching, teenagers become more proficient in the skills and knowledge they share. What jumps out as a quintessential example of this is when Noah started teaching the beginners' kids class at our BJJ school. He quickly realized there were new levels of his own understanding to be unlocked just the instant he was bombarded with an array of questions he had never considered before about the very simple arm bar he himself had learned on HIS first day of class. Obviously, he knew how to perform the move, I have seen him execute it in competition dozens of times, and this does not count the thousand repetitions we have put in during our daily drilling over the past three years. AND YET... when a 6 year old asked, "Where do I put my thumb? Does it matter which hand I use?"

Noah found himself looking over to me, not 100% sure of whether or not that intricacy had any impact on the efficacy of the technique.

Needless to say, Noah developed a firmer grasp (no pun intended) of the nuances and intricacies of this subject matter, enabling him to approach it with more significant expertise. By deepening their understanding and mastery, teenagers solidify their own foundation of knowledge and become more confident in their abilities.

Enhancing Communication and Interpersonal Skills: Teaching and training others provides teenagers with valuable opportunities to enhance their communication and interpersonal skills. As they convey information and ideas to others, they must learn to articulate their thoughts clearly, adapt their communication style to different audiences, and engage effectively with their listeners.

By practicing effective communication, teenagers develop their ability to express themselves with clarity, brevity, and relevance. They learn to listen actively, observe non-verbal cues, and tailor their communication to ensure understanding. These skills not only benefit their teaching and training endeavors but also transfer to other areas of their lives, enabling them to communicate more effectively in personal and professional relationships.

Fostering Empathy and Compassion: In case it hasn't registered quite yet, I hope we have adequately demonstrated the concept that with regard to these chapters and the ideas contained therein, one hand washes the other, so to speak. Each leadership quality you internalize and improve at vastly strengthens your capacity to execute all the others. This chapter is no exception. Teaching others fosters empathy and compassion within teenagers. As they step into the role of educators, they must understand their learners' needs, challenges, and perspectives. This requires them to empathize with their audience and tailor their teachings to address their unique circumstances.

Through teaching and training, teenagers develop a heightened sense of empathy as they consider the learning styles, strengths, and limitations of their mentees. They become more attuned to the emotions and needs of others, fostering a compassionate and supportive environment for learning. By cultivating empathy and compassion, teenagers develop an essential quality of influential leaders who can understand and connect with those they lead.

Teaching and training others allow teenagers to leave a lasting impact on the lives of those they educate. By sharing their knowledge and expertise, they contribute to the growth, development, and success of their mentees. They become catalysts for positive change, empowering others to reach their full potential.

Through teaching and training, teenagers become part of a more extensive legacy of knowledge sharing. They pass on their insights and experiences, ensuring that their contributions continue to make a difference even beyond their immediate interactions. By leaving a lasting impact, teenagers become influential leaders who inspire and empower others to embrace their own leadership journeys. Passing on a part of themselves, even after they are no longer present with that person or group, and thus achieving, according to the Dalai Lama, their own preverbal immortality.

Final Thoughts On Sharing Knowledge

Someone probably significantly smarter than I am once said, "Great leaders don't create followers, they create other leaders."

I believe this to be perhaps the final stage, if there was one, in the maturation of the leadership process. As teenagers share their knowledge, they contribute to the development of future leaders. By nurturing the skills and talents of others, they lay the foundation for a generation of capable and confident individuals who are equipped to take on leadership roles in various domains. The impact of their teachings extends far beyond their immediate circle as the knowledge they share continues to spread and shape the world around them.

They become catalysts for change, igniting a thirst for knowledge, inspiring curiosity, and fostering growth in themselves and others. By recognizing the importance of teaching and training, teenagers embark on a journey of self-discovery, transformation, and making a positive impact on the world.

Embracing The Journey

Parenting is already a tough job - it's like being a manager, therapist, and chef all in one. But it's worth it because we want our kids to thrive and be successful.

We've covered a lot of ground in this book, from building confidence, teamwork to time management, from gratitude to goal setting. These are all essential skills for leaders, and by teaching them to your teen, you're setting them up for success in all areas of their life.

But let's not kid ourselves - raising a leader is a lifelong journey. There will be ups and downs, twists and turns, and probably a few meltdowns along the way (both for you and your teen). But that's okay, because it's all part of the process. Embrace the journey and enjoy the ride. And who knows, maybe your teen will even teach you a thing or two about leadership along the way.

I know some of these strategies may seem daunting or even downright impossible to implement at first. But trust me when I say that all the effort you put into cultivating leadership in your teenager will be well worth it in the long run. Being a leader is not just about being the boss or barking orders left and right. It's about being a role model and inspiring others to bring their A-game. By fostering leadership in your teenager, you're giving them the tools they need to make a real difference in their communities, schools, and workplaces.

It's a continual process that requires a whole lot of patience, dedication, and perseverance. It may take some time for your teenager to fully embrace their leadership potential, still, with your unwavering guidance and support, they'll get there eventually.

So, I urge you to take what you have learned from this book and begin implementing these strategies in your daily life. Talk to your teenager about their goals and aspirations, and work with them to develop a plan to achieve them.

I know it can be tough to raise a teenager, and there will be times when you feel like throwing in the towel. But trust me, you're not the only one who feels that way. Every parent goes through their own set of challenges, whether it's dealing with teenage mood swings or navigating social media trends. So, don't be afraid to reach out for help when you need it.

You could ask other parents for advice, hit up professionals who have seen it all, or even ask your own teenager for some insight. They might just surprise you with their perspective. And who knows, maybe they'll even give you a pointer or two on how to handle their teenage behavior.

Remember, it's not a sign of weakness to ask for help. In fact, it takes real strength to admit when you need a hand.

So, don't be afraid to lean on your support system. After all, it takes a village to raise a teenager!

But don't forget, raising leaders isn't just about developing skills and qualities in your teenager. It's also about being a role model and practicing what you preach. You can't expect your teen to be a great leader if you're not leading by example.

Take the time to evaluate your own leadership skills and qualities.

Do you possess the same qualities that you wish to instill in your child? Are you effectively communicating with them, making sound decisions, and managing your time wisely? Are you promoting their independence, fostering a positive mindset, and encouraging collaboration? Your child looks up to you, and leading by example is one of the most potent ways to influence their behavior.

As we know, parenting is a journey, and there will be bumps in the road. It won't always be smooth sailing. There will be challenges and obstacles along the way, and it's normal to feel overwhelmed or unsure at times. However, if you stay committed to implementing the fifteen strategies we've discussed in this book and approach your role as a parent with intention and purpose, you can help your teenager develop into a leader who is confident, capable, and compassionate.

This vast undertaking does not warrant a one-size-fits-all approach. What works for one family may not work for another. So, be flexible and adaptable with these strategies.

Some may require more effort and time than others. Some may be resisted or rejected by your teen entirely. Stay the course. I assure you, This Juice is worth the squeeze. More so, in fact, than any other sweetness I have experienced in my time here on earth. Being proud of the man my son is, turbulent as the process became through points, has been the most rewarding experience in my life.

So, take a deep breath, enjoy the ride, and trust yourself. Trust yourself to be the leader for your teen to model after. Trust in your instincts that you know what to do. Where to push and where to pull. For the times that you are in over your head, and you truly don't know the answer; I have one more piece of wisdom to impart.

Ironically, I'd like to conclude our exploration of leadership and parenting with a trip back to the very beginning of my parenting journey.

Afterword: A Not-So-Quick Word About Having Faith

When we first found out we were having Noah, my wife and I were on our "Honeymoon," aka a semester abroad program called "Semester at Sea." Very accurate to the title of the program, SAS was essentially 500 ish college kids circumnavigating the globe on a partially converted cruise ship containing certain floors, or "decks", that bore a very vague and distant resemblance to a university campus where we would attend classes in between ports.

Sea sickness was quite common, especially while in rough patches of the ocean, like rounding the tip of the caped horn of South Africa. So, when Heidi was throwing up, it was simply par for the course. When her cycle was off, this wasn't uncommon either, apparently, and we chalked it up to the same thing many of the other young women were attributing these phenomena to, which was eating weird foods, having erratic sleeping hours, and introducing the body to a myriad of new medications for each new country we visited to stay compliant with their customs requirements.

By the time we disembarked in Chennai, India, Heidi was STILL vomiting profusely and almost a month late. I put my foot down, and we went to get a pregnancy test from a third-world pharmacy… a feat not to be brushed over lightly, as there was not a single word of common language shared between us and the Indian pharmacist.

In fact, even the non-verbal head shake customarily used to indicate "no" was different. Instead of rotating the head, pointing your nose at one shoulder, then turning and pointing your nose at the other shoulder back and forth to indicate "no", it was more of a tilting of the head one ear to one shoulder then the other ear to the other shoulder in sort of a bobble motion. I don't mean that disparagingly, I've just simply never been put in the position to describe a head nod or shake, let alone one of a different culture that may be less intuitive an image to somebody who has never witnessed it.

Nevertheless, we eventually obtained the baby stick of fortune and missioned behind the decaying building of a pharmacy, making sure to avoid any rusted structures, or wildly roaming cattle to what we were moderately sure we were told was their bathroom. Pretty much a wooden plank to provide at least one direction of privacy, and a hole in the ground. Squatting like the well-assimilated sari-wearing tourist and soon-to-be mother she was, Heidi tinkles over the stick. A few minutes later, sure as shit, at 20 years old, halfway around the world in a foreign culture with only a few Rupees to my name (which is saying a lot because I believe at the time, they were like 1400 to 1 with the US Dollar), we find out, bum bum da da! It's mothatruckin' baby time.

Speechless, and terrified, Heidi looks up at me with eyes silently pleading, "Say something".

In a falsely nonchalant tone (improvisational as it was, it seemed to be effective in masking my own panic while simultaneously easing my wife's worry), I smiled and said the first thing that came to my mind: "Well, seeing as we are on a ship going around the world... boy or girl, I think we should name them Noah."

We laughed and hugged. Excited, relieved, in shock, and quite frankly, scared shitless.

"Seriously Joshua, wtf are we going to do?" Heidi questioned me in what was at the time still a very thick accent from Manchester, England.

"Well, if it's a girl, we can drop the 'H'. Maybe just Noa." I obfuscated humorously.

"I'm being serious!" She exclaims, swatting my arm. A gentle indication she was running out of patience for my usual way of handling stressful scenarios with humor deflections. Still a shortcoming I am working on to this day.

I took a deep breath and asked the universe for guidance. My initial thought was to comment on the fact that we were sitting in a field next to a pit someone dug and called it a restroom, but my better self grabbed the wheel instead;

"You know Heidi, I don't have a super clear game plan, but we'll make one. I don't know why, or where it's coming from, but I have this overwhelming faith that we'll learn how to be parents, and we'll figure it out. Piece by piece, one step and one day at a time as we go."

She looked up at me like, "Who are you, and what have you done with my mischievous shithead of a husband" but apparently, those words, wherever they came from, were exactly what we both needed to hear...

What activated in me? Cosmic insight, answering my silent plea of "Holy hell, what are we going to do"? Evolutionary cellular intelligence that just turns on when you find out you're becoming a parent?

Or was it that deep down inside of us, below the jaded worldview, below the egoic self-aggrandizing assimilation of events, we convince ourselves to secure our position in a big scary world, below whatever resentments we hold toward one traditional religion or another... there is a knowingness.

A knowingness that there is something larger at play here. A guiding force of some kind. If the word God is too touchy, try something else. Fate? Karma? Wayne Dyer used to call it "source." Russel Brand refers to it as the sacred.

I do not profess to understand this force, heck, I don't even have an exact name for it. Which, as I am writing this seems rather silly and inappropriate that an all-powerful, incomprehensible, and pervasive force would require such a reductive classification as a human word. Words can be great, but let's be honest, at certain times, with certain things, they are deeply insufficient.

It's why I hesitated to even write a chapter on faith and, against my own internal insecurity, decided to take a crack at it anyway. So instead of making an intellectual or verbal argument for what I personally believe this guiding higher power to be, I will say this… It is imperative we have one.

We need it in times we straight up do not know what to do or how to handle something. Like, say, I don't know, the reality adjustment of finding out I'm prematurely going to be a parent. When our intellect and experience fall short, we need to be able to surrender to the knowingness (not just intellectually but the secure FEELING of knowing) that something's got our back and all we got to do is our part, as hard as we can do it.

And, well, to stay semi-on-track with the story without getting too esoteric or nebulous… that's what I did. What I perceived to be my part, as hard as I could do it. I finished out semester at sea. I came home, loaded up on units (I took 23 and 21 my last two semesters at school), and started my first business helping homeowners recover money for the cleanup of smoke, soot, and ash after wildfires. Of course, it didn't hurt that the very year I embarked on this endeavor, San Diego had one of the largest wildfires in California's history, leaving plenty of people to be helped.

Andrew Carnegie said, in order to become wildly successful, you need brains, balls, and a couple of lucky breaks… I definitely think my first brush with entrepreneurial success was way more lucky break being in the right place at the right time than it was brains or balls, but that notwithstanding, my life was, although quite difficult, starting to take shape. My faith seemed to be well founded.

Never really sleeping more than 3-4 hours per night with a brand-new infant, relying heavily on babysitting points from my mother when possible, taking over double what constituted a full load in school, and starting a business, I was quite overwhelmed.

Not sure if I was going to be able to push through to the end of school to graduate, I found it remarkable when I heard Steve Jobs, a dude that dropped out of college, had been awarded an honorary doctorate degree, and was the premier speaker for the Stanford graduation ceremony.

I watched the video of the speech he gave without exaggeration thousands of times. It moved me deeply. So much so, in fact, I would watch it every morning on YouTube right when I woke up before I would do anything. I can still probably recite most of it by heart. In his speech, he told three stories. The following is one of them I'd like to share with you about faith (a word he would never have used), or what he calls "connecting the dots":

Steve Jobs Stanford Commencement Speech:

"CONNECTING THE DOTS

The first story is about connecting the dots. I dropped out of Reed College after the first 6 months, but then stayed around as a drop-in for another 18 months or so before I really quit.

So why did I drop out?

It started before I was born. My biological mother was a young, unwed graduate student, and she decided to put me up for adoption. She felt very strongly that I should be adopted by college graduates, so everything was all set for me to be adopted at birth by a lawyer and his wife.

Except that when I popped out, they decided at the last minute that they really wanted a girl.

So my parents, who were on a waiting list, got a call in the middle of the night asking: "We've got an unexpected baby boy; do you want him?"

They said: "Of course."

When my biological mother found out later that my mother had never graduated from college and that my father had never graduated from high school. She refused to sign the final adoption papers. She only relented a few months later when my parents promised that I would go to college.

This was the start in my life.

And 17 years later, I did go to college. But I naively chose a college that was almost as expensive as Stanford, and all of my working-class parents' savings were being spent on my college tuition.

After six months, I couldn't see the value in it. I had no idea what I wanted to do with my life or how college would help me figure it out.

And here I was, spending all of the money my parents had saved their entire life. So I decided to drop out and trust that it would all work out OK.

It was pretty scary at the time, but looking back, it was one of the best decisions I ever made.

The minute I dropped out, I could stop taking the required classes that didn't interest me and begin dropping in on the ones that looked far more interesting.

It wasn't all romantic. I didn't have a dorm room, so I slept on the floor in friends' rooms, I returned coke bottles for the $0.05 deposits to buy food with, and I would walk the 7 miles across town every Sunday night to get one good meal a week at the Hare Krishna temple. I loved it.

And much of what I stumbled into by following my curiosity and intuition turned out to be priceless later on.

Let me give you one example: Reed College, at that time, offered perhaps the best calligraphy instruction in the country. Throughout the campus, every poster, and every label on every drawer, was beautifully hand calligraphed.

Because I had dropped out and didn't have to take the normal classes, I decided to take a calligraphy class to learn how to do this. I learned about serif and san serif typefaces, about varying the amount of space between different letter combinations, and about what makes great typography great.

It was beautiful, historical, and artistically subtle in a way that science can't capture, and I found it fascinating.

None of this had even a hope of any practical application in my life.

But 10 years later, when we were designing the first Macintosh computer, it all came back to me. And we designed it all into the Mac. It was the first computer with beautiful typography.

If I had never dropped in on that single course in college, the Mac would have never had multiple typefaces or proportionally spaced fonts. And since Windows just copied the Mac, it's likely that no personal computer would have them.

If I had never dropped out, I would have never dropped in on this calligraphy class, and personal computers might not have the wonderful typography that they do.

Of course, it was impossible to connect the dots looking forward when I was in college. But it was very, very clear looking backward 10 years later.

Again, you can't connect the dots looking forward; you can only connect them looking backward.

So you have to trust that the dots will somehow connect in your future. You have to trust in something — your gut, destiny, life, karma, whatever.

Because believing that the dots will connect down the road will give you the confidence to follow your heart even when it leads you off the well-worn path, and that will make all the difference."

Although Steve Jobs used the words "trust" in things like "your gut, destiny, life, karma," ... if this is not a masterful depiction of the same exact phenomena I referred to as "faith," I don't know what is. The words don't matter as much as the principle belief in something you cannot yet see, smell, taste, touch, or fully conceive.

I used to believe perception is reality. The truth is, that is ragingly short-sighted. The limit of our perception is undoubtedly NOT the limit of reality or all that exists… that's ludicrous. That is like standing on your roof looking at the horizon, proclaiming that where your sight stops, the world stops!

Of course, we know better. We know that our sight, or capacity to visually perceive, is limited. We also know that if we were to move a mile in the direction of our line of sight, our ability to perceive (aka our vision) would extend a mile further in that direction. It would be absurd to say that where our perception ends, the world ends.

The same is true with the nature of reality. We can only see but a fraction of the spectrum of light. Yet, with instrumentation, we know that a greater array of light exists.

We readily accept there are frequencies of sounds we can't hear, but dogs can. Do we doubt the "noise" coming out of a dog whistle exists? Of course, we don't, whether or not it is imperceptible to us.

Why is it so difficult for us to, at times, apply the same degree of latitude or logical grace to the concept that there may be invisible forces at work gently (or, in my case, not so gently at times) guiding us? Even as I'm writing this, I hear my intellect's protestations; "So you just want me to just blindly accept inconceivable, invisible forces are intelligently at work, even though we lack any concrete evidence"?

Just as reality is not limited by our capacity to perceive in the form of sight or sound, so is it not limited by our limited capacity to understand? Said inversely, there is more to reality than simply what we can understand about reality. If you require hard evidence of inexplicable yet undeniable intelligence, you need look no further than coral. While I may be writing this overlooking Kaanapali beach in Maui, what brings this to mind is actually an episode of the Joe Rogan Experience Podcast. Here's a rough quote of what I just heard:

"The secret behind coral's telepathic communication - every year on the same day at the same hour within the same minute, corals of the same species, although separated by thousands of miles, will suddenly spawn with perfect synchronicity.

The dates and times vary from year to year for reasons only the coral knows.

While one species of coral spawns during one hour, another species right next to it waits for a different hour or different day, or different week to spawn in synchronicity with its own species.

Distance seems to have no effect. If you broke off a chunk of coral and placed it in a bucket beneath a sink in London, that chunk WOULD spawn at the same time as other coral of that species around the world....

Coral is the largest biological structure on the planet and covers 175 thousand miles of the sea floor. It can clearly communicate far more sophisticatedly than anyone ever thought. And yet, it is one of the most primitive "animals" on earth. Coral has no eyes, no ears, and no brain."

No eyes, no ears, and no brain. Yet, it contains intelligence. An observable intelligence and design, even unity, that we can't fully explain. Shit, aside from fumbling around with clumsy words like "telepathy", we can't in good conscience even pretend to partially explain this phenomenon. Such is true with the current that is guiding our lives.

Especially those of us with a propensity for analysis, an above-average intellect, or overly exercised "logic muscle," so to speak, pride ourselves in our capacity to intellectually wrestle with the concept of faith. Of surrendering to the inevitable fact that just as there are levels of light we can't see, and sound we can't hear, there's intelligence we can't explain, or dare I say it, even conceive of.

But just because reality is not limited simply by our capacity to understand, that doesn't mean that we can't harness this truth for our own (and universal) benefit.

It is my contention that there are no atheists in foxholes, as it were. With bullets whizzing by your head in a war zone, you would be hard-pressed to not plead toward SOMETHING for safety or protection. If, God forbid (excusing the expression), you heard news of a very close immediate relative or loved one being in a severe accident of some kind, self-proclaimed agnostic or not, it'd be challenging to not find yourself saying, "Please let them be ok."

What exactly are we petitioning for safety while in the depths of fear and adrenaline, clutching our weapons and facing what could be our imminent demise? Who or what are we asking for protection over a loved one when notified that they could potentially not be ok? We don't need a definitive or descriptive answer for that inquiry other than a simple internal acknowledgment that we are asking.

We are petitioning something. Requesting protection (using the aforementioned examples) from something. I offer the supposition that this "Something" is, in fact, the very same intelligence guiding corals' capacity to perform magic tricks. The same intelligence that makes our fingernails grow. The same thing we know is there but sometimes requires desperation in order to connect with.

The very same universe a 20-year-old would "pray" to, for lack of a better word, in a field on his ass, minutes after finding out he's gonna be a dad for the first time.

I would never be so presumptuous or cavalier as to presume I have the capacity to explain this force in its entirety, but what I can tell you is that at least from my own personal experience, when I have the willingness to acknowledge its existence and generate the humility and willingness to surrender my inevitable inadequacies to it… it will carry us.

We will no longer resist the tide or create pain and friction caused by our desire to control. Instead, this force, that I believe to be guiding us anyway, whether or not we surrender to the fact it exists, can more effortlessly flow us upon the universal current toward the uncharacteristically perfect words when we previously had none.

The current that can drift us toward our first job that is more about the right place at the right time, than it is about individual brilliance. Toward the typography class that later leads to personal computers containing the function of fonts a decade later. The force that can guide a scared, barely self-sufficient 20-year-old twirp, toward self-belief and courage, through a sequence of events he would not have had the capacity to design himself in 10,000 lifetimes despite what my ego tells me at times.

A divine and brutal sequence that starts in a field in Chennai, India, and continues until that very same protagonist finds himself faced with the previously unfathomable prospect of writing a parenting book. The intelligence that does, always has, and always most certainly will make the dots connect.

Generally speaking, especially those of us with a propensity toward going all-in on the things we are passionate about, run the risk of "over-parenting" our teens. Especially when we are either worried about them in some capacity, or after having read a wildly stimulating parenting book filled with incredible suggestions and a slew of new exercises and techniques to beef up our parenting game has us all excited.

If you find yourself rip, rearing, and ready to rock... about to re-do your future leader's entire schedule and use all these new tactics all at once, let me save you some trouble with this sage advice: don't. Breathe into your tummy. Then exhale, and believe me when I tell you that you will find way better results with a deeper internalization of these concepts and a slow implementation (while ensuring to read your audience and gauge the feedback your teen is giving you) than you will by implementing the inverse.

To that point, Dr. Russell Barkley, an internationally recognized authority on the subject of parenting children with ADHD, illustrates a magnificent argument as to why, as parents, overreaching or micromanaging can be a task in utter futility. The following is an excerpt from a speech he gave almost a decade ago that can still be found on YouTube and is very much worth the watch:

"You need to understand something the parents these days have long since forgotten and are going to have to relearn. Again, your grandparents knew this, but today's generation of parents doesn't seem to, and that is... You do not get to design your children!

Nature would never have permitted that to happen. Evolution would not have allowed a generation of a species to be so influenced by the previous generation. It hasn't happened, and it doesn't happen, and it especially doesn't happen in children. You do not design your children, and yet we have the Mozart effect.

The belief is that if I play classical music to my uterus when I'm pregnant, I will have a genius! If I can just put enough crib toys over his crib, he will have all these neurons exploding with synapses and be a brilliant mathematician! You don't get that degree of power.

Does that mean stimulation doesn't matter? No, it means a stimulating environment is better than a deprived environment, but it doesn't mean that the more stimulation you add to the environment, the better. But it gets to a threshold where there is enough stimulation that every normal brain needs to develop, and once you're past that, which 98 of you are, the rest of it is out of your hands.

But this idea that if a little bit is good, a ton of it must be better is a uniquely North American perspective.

So, what we have learned in the last 20 years of research in neuroimaging, Behavior, genetics, developmental psychology, and neuropsychology can be boiled down to this phrase:

Your child is born with more than 400 psychological traits that will emerge as they mature, and THEY HAVE NOTHING TO DO WITH YOU.

So the idea that you are going to engineer personalities, IQ, academic achievement skills, and all these other things just isn't accurate. Your child is not a blank slate on which you get to write. If you would like to read more about this, please read Steven Pinker's book "The Blank Slate," which reviews all of this information for parents and why it isn't true.

The better view is that your child is a genetic mosaic of your extended family. This means a unique combination of the traits that run in your family line. I like the shepherd's view; You are a shepherd. You don't design the sheep.

The engineering view makes you responsible for everything. Everything that goes right and everything that goes wrong. This is why parents come to us with such guilt! More guilt than we've ever seen in Prior Generations because parents today believe that it's all about them, and what they do. And, if they don't get it right or if their child has a disability, they've done something wrong when in fact, the opposite is true. This has nothing to do with your particular brand of parenting.

I would rather that you stop thinking of yourself as an engineer and step back and say, "I am a Shepherd" to a unique individual. Shepherds are powerful people! They pick the pastures in which the Sheep will graze and develop and grow.

They determine whether they're appropriately nourished. They've determined whether they're protected from harm. The environment is important, but it doesn't design the Sheep. No Shepherd is going to turn a sheep into a dog! Ain't gonna happen, right? And that is what we see parents trying to do all the time! Especially parents of children with disabilities. So step back and view yourself as the shepherd to this youngster, and you get to design the pasture, and that it's very important, but you don't engineer the Sheep.

Now that comes with it, a profoundly freeing view of parenting because what it means is although it's important to be a shepherd, recognizing that this is a unique individual BEFORE YOU allows you to enjoy the show!

So open a bottle of Chardonnay, kick off your slippers, sit back, and watch what takes place because you don't get to determine this. So just enjoy it! It doesn't last all that long, anyway. They're gone before you know it!

If you think that what you did in your house is going to shape the life course of this individual, you are sadly mistaken. This is a unique individual. Let them grow. Let them Prosper. Please design appropriate environments around them, but you don't get to design them.

As Judy Harris said in 1996 in the first book on this subject written for laypeople, the book is called the nurture assumption, as she said, you have more to do with your child's life by where you choose to live than by anything you will ever do inside that home short of abuse, neglect, or malnutrition. The rest of it is just a trivial variation.

It's where you live. Why? Because out-of-home influences are more powerful in shaping your child's life course than in-home influences are. Those out-of-home influences are peer groups, other adults, neighborhoods, resources, schools, and the larger community that you made available to this child. That is how you shape your child's life course.

The second most significant influence is also out of your hands, and that's genetics. You don't get to determine that, but if you think parenting is so influential, let me give you two findings that have been replicated many times.

When we follow up with twins, we are able to calculate how much of their behavior is due to parenting within the family environment, and here's what we find. The peak years of parental influence are below seven! From seven on to 12, it drops dramatically. After 15, it's six percent. Six percent of the variation in a teenager's behavior is how their parents raise them. That's it. After age 21, it's zero. Parenting has no influence on any psychological trait after the age of 21.

Now, do not mistake what I'm saying. The knowledge your child possesses, what they know is clearly a function of exposure in the environment but their traits, their abilities, their makeup, their personality is not."

So why the hell give you this? Why have you spent hours reading what took me months of writing, getting you all juiced up on a new approach (or at least providing you with what are presumably some decently interesting perspectives), only to then turn around and tell you that your impact is marginal (ONLY 6% according to this study) past a certain stage?

The answer is twofold:

Number one, to whatever degree we CAN influence our children positively, we should.

And two, to the extent we CAN'T, we get to release our grasp and enjoy the ride.

To the extent we CAN create a difference…

I don't care if the influence on my son's psyche, capacity for happiness, or psychological well-being was only 1%… I would fight with everything I have for that 1% improvement. Wouldn't you? As I stated earlier… that juice is worth the squeeze. It reminds me of another highly inspirational speech from a movie, Any Given Sunday. Admittedly, a film whose overall quality I can't quite attest to, as its been many years since I've watched it. What I can say is that Al Pachino's halftime speech as the coach of a fictional football team was world-class.

Here it is:

"I don't know what to say, really. Three minutes to the biggest battle of our professional lives, all comes down to today. Either we heal as a team, or we're going to crumble, inch by inch, play by play, 'til we're finished.

We're in hell right now, gentlemen, believe me. And we can stay here, get the shit kicked out of us, or we can fight our way back into the light. We can climb out of hell, one inch at a time. Now I can't do it for you. I'm too old. I look around, I see these young faces, and I think, I mean, I made every wrong choice a middle-aged man can make.

I pissed away all my money, believe it or not. I chased off anyone who's ever loved me, and lately, I can't even stand the face I see in the mirror. You know, when you get old in life, things get taken from you. I mean, that's part of life. But you only learn that when you start losing stuff.

You find out life's this game of inches. So is football because, in either game, life or football, the margin for error is so small. I mean, one half a step too late or too early, and you don't quite make it. One half second, too slow, too fast, you don't quite catch it. The inches we need are everywhere around us.

They're in every game break, minute, and second. On this team, we fight for that inch. On this team, we tear ourselves and everyone else around us to pieces for that inch. We claw with our fingernails for that inch because we know when we add up all those inches, that's going to make the fucking difference between winning and losing, between living and dying.

I'll tell you this, in any fight, it's the guy who's willing to die, who will win that inch. And I know if I'm going to have any life anymore, it's because I'm still willing to fight and die for that inch because that's what living is, the six inches in front of your face. Now I can't make you do it. You got to look at the guy next to you, look into his eyes.

Now I think you're going to see a guy who will go that inch with you. You're going to see a guy who will sacrifice himself for this team because he knows when it comes down to it, you're going to do the same for him. That's a team, gentlemen. And either we heal now as a team, or we will die as individuals. That's life. That's football, guys. That's all it is. Now, what are you going to do?"

Man! Reading that still gets me pumped! I mean, how perfect? The game might be life, not football. The team may be a family, not a sports team. I may not have chased off everyone that loves me or made every wrong decision a middle-aged man can make, but… ok fine, maybe it's not a PERFECT parallel, but the common threads still run pretty deep.

I mean, on a sports team, one player can't make every pass and every catch. One lineman can't hit the block AND be the one carrying the ball. What they, and we, CAN do is our part. As hard as we can. For ourselves and our teammates… primarily our children. As is the case in this metaphor, we can inspire our family with our actions, fighting for the inch of difference we actually CAN make, which in turn, encourages them to do the same. And life, according to a fictional football coach, has me reliving my glory days as team captain of a division 3, private school, 8-man high school football team… is simply a game of inches.

To the extent that we CAN NOT make a difference-

Either because the circumstances don't fit the genetic coding of our loved one, they have a different ideal they are attempting to adhere to, or the play simply isn't ours to carry out… WE MUST LEARN TO RELEASE CONTROL. Surrender is one of these paradoxical things, right? In the 12 steps of AA, as soon as one surrenders, "admitting they are powerless" over whatever their addiction of choice is… they become endowed with a capacity to start influencing their lives again towards sobriety. To the extent we relinquish domineering or controlling patterns over strong-willed family members, loved ones, or co-workers… the more we see their innate willingness to hear and receive our input.

Teens, and to a certain extent all people, can be a tricky beast in this capacity. Much like sand, if we summon the ability to just hold it in our hand, it will stay there. If we squeeze too hard out of a desire for it not to leave us, it will run through our fingers. I'm not saying if you squeeze your teen, they're going to run away (hell, Noah and I choke each other constantly while training, and my mom still squeezes me as hard as she can, giving awkwardly long hugs to this day) but, what I am saying, is there is a great power in releasing the forcefulness with which we are showing our love and guidance.

When I am able to connect with the fact that the influence I am having by his teenage years is only 6% (allegedly anyway), and therefore inversely, the influence I am NOT having is 94%... I can just chill. I can be there if he needs me without pounding on him to hear my unsolicited advice.

I can hear him out as his own person. I can sit back in absolute friggin' awe of this beautiful gift in the form of a being that I realize I played a part in manifesting but did not create in his entirety. He, like myself, is many things. Not just one. I can surrender to the fact that life passed through me and into him.

He is not my creation but my teammate, my buddy, my student, and my teacher. I sit back and look at the fact that he is me. The closest I've ever gotten to consciously being able to connect with the "Buddha mind" or the unification of all things is in recognition of the deep invisible yet palpable connection between us guised in the illusion of separation. I am re-having this existential epiphany…

And then, he goes, "Dad, C'mon … can we bounce? You're staring at me like a weirdo, and we're late for practice!". Hah, and I'm right back to realizing there ARE still things I can do to foster the proper environment, make sure he is protected, stimulated, and by the time I am done here… a deeply self-sufficient and profoundly impactful leader.

Thanks for reading.

Joshua Nussbaum

Your Journey Matters

Thank you for investing your time in reading this book.

Your opinion matters to me greatly. I kindly request you to leave a review for this book, sharing your experience, learning, and the way it might have influenced your approach towards leadership and parenting.

Your feedback will not only help me improve my future content, but it will also assist other parents in choosing resources that can help them in their journey towards raising confident, empathetic, and resilient teenagers.

To leave a review, please scan the QR code below.

Once again, we thank you for your time and support.

Made in United States
Orlando, FL
12 August 2023

35994304R00152